I0518358

FINDING HOPE & JOY IN CANCER

WISDOM FOR PATIENTS, CAREGIVERS, FAMILY & FRIENDS

AMANDA GUNVILLE

The stories and reflections in this book come from the author's own journey with cancer. They are shared to offer encouragement, comfort, and hope. Nothing in these pages should replace the guidance of your doctors, care team, or other licensed professionals.

Finding Hope & Joy in Cancer: Wisdom for Patients, Caregivers, Family & Friends
Copyright © 2025 by Amanda Gunville

All rights reserved.
Published by Hope & Joy LLC

This book is licensed for your personal enjoyment only. It may not be resold, copied, or shared without the author's permission, except for brief quotations used in reviews or articles.

ISBN: 979-8-9999218-1-9
eBook ISBN: 979-8-9999218-0-2

Printed in the United States of America

For more information, visit: www.HopeAndJoy.net

Dedication:

To my family—
You were my anchor, my comic relief, my tireless chauffeurs, and my fiercest advocates. Mom, Dad, Brother, my husband, and my sweet daughter—you carried me when I couldn't carry myself and reminded me that love is the best medicine.

And to *Amanda's Army*—
My circle of warriors, care package senders, prayer givers, texters, meal deliverers, cheerleaders, and quiet hand-holders. You proved an army doesn't need uniforms—it can show up with book recommendations, casseroles, hugs, playlists, and inappropriate jokes at just the right moment.

This book belongs to you as much as it does to me.

Introduction

When I was first diagnosed with stage 2, triple-positive breast cancer, I was desperate for answers, for control, for hope. I did what any overachieving, Type-A person would do when faced with a life-altering diagnosis: I tried to out-research the disease. I ordered every book I could find on how to beat cancer. I signed up for online courses. I booked virtual appointments with integrative oncologists across the country. I scoured studies, podcasts, and survivor blogs, and even clicked on the spam ad that offered to cure me with kale and goat yoga. My days—and many sleepless nights—were filled with attempts to decode the science, piece together protocols, and build the perfect plan to survive.

And while the resources I found were well-researched and full of expertise, they were also long, overly technical, and, at times, filled with fear-based messaging. They were often written in a tone best described as "clinical robot with a PhD in fear." I would start each book with good intentions, but quickly find myself overwhelmed and emotionally drained. What I needed wasn't another academic dissertation. I needed wisdom fast—something accessible, digestible, and grounded in real-life experience. I didn't need to be scared into change. The worst had already happened.

So, I learned on the go. I learned while hooked up to IVs. I learned in waiting rooms. I learned in quiet moments with my daughter asleep next to me, and I learned through hard conversations with my family, doctors, and—most importantly—myself. And somewhere along the way, I found my rhythm. I found a plan. Not a perfect one, but one that worked for me—one that was both scientific and spiritual, both structured and intuitive.

Since then, I've had many friends reach out to ask if I'd speak with someone newly diagnosed or in the thick of treatment. It always starts with the same text: "I hate to ask, but would you talk to my friend?" And my answer is always YES. Because once you've walked this path, you don't let others walk it alone. Those women (and sometimes men) are now part of a club none of us ever wanted to join, but one I now fiercely honor. They are my fellow warriors. And with each call, each walk-and-talk, each shared tear and laugh, I realized: maybe this wasn't just *my* experience. Perhaps it was meant to be shared.

Several therapists and friends gently nudged me to write. A book. A blog. A social media page. Anything. I always shrugged it off—I'm not a writer. But then one night, I woke up with a start, and the words were already there. I grabbed my phone, opened the Notes app, and started typing like I was taking dictation from the universe. From then on, I wrote only when inspired, often outside, surrounded by nature with the sun or stars above me and the wind at my back.

This book was born from those moments. It's not a textbook or a treatment manual. It's part memoir, part guidebook, and part coffee-with-a-friend-who's-been-through-it-and-will-tell-you-the-truth-but-still-make-you-laugh. Inside, you'll find the words, mindsets, and tools that not only helped me through treatment but also helped me radically transform my life into something better than it was before cancer. My hope is that it inspires you, makes you laugh, maybe cry, and most of all, reminds you that you're not alone.

The beginning chapters share what my life looked like before cancer hit—the pace, habits, and pressures that shaped me leading up to my diagnosis. Maybe you'll recognize some of those same patterns in your own life—and if so, let my story serve as a gentle warning, a chance to make changes before life insists on it.

You'll also find the unfiltered truth of what cancer looks like up close—the fear, the frustration, the heartbreak—but also the small sparks of joy that can change everything. Some chapters are raw, some are tender, and some may make you laugh when you least expect it. Together, they paint a picture of what it means to not only survive, but to live fully—even in the middle of the unthinkable.

If I could hand you a cup of tea (or a glass of wine—your call) and sit with you on the couch to walk you through what helped me—not just to survive, but to slowly and intentionally rebuild a joyful, vibrant life—this would be that conversation.

Welcome.

Chapter 1: The Call

"Life changes in the instant. The ordinary instant." — Joan Didion

It started as an ordinary day—the kind that doesn't hint at any shift in the ground beneath your feet.

I was in the kitchen, one hand on my phone, the other juggling the chaos that comes with raising a toddler. My daughter was eighteen months old—a walking, babbling hurricane of energy —and I was running on adrenaline most days. I hadn't had time to schedule my annual OB/GYN exam since her birth, mainly since we no longer lived in Arizona, where she was born. But I needed a refill on my birth control, so I called my old doctor in Phoenix.

She refused.

No refill without an updated exam.

I sighed. There was no way I was risking an accidental baby number two. I was tired—deep-in-my-bones tired—and I couldn't even wrap my mind around the idea of being pregnant again. So, I made an appointment at a local clinic and went in, not thinking much of it beyond getting what I needed and getting back to my life.

The appointment was routine. Standard questions. Cold exam table. Then, as she wrapped up, the doctor mentioned I was overdue for a mammogram. I was 41, already a year late.

That simple reminder shifted something in me. I remembered 2012, the lump I'd found, the biopsy that turned out to be benign cystic tissue. That scare had landed me on a cycle of mammograms every six months for a while, but eventually, things normalized, and I got cleared. Still, her words stuck.

Later that day, I scheduled the mammogram.

I even joked with the tech when I went in. She had kind eyes and a calming demeanor. We laughed about how mammograms are the worst best part of turning 40—necessary, uncomfortable, but oddly bonding. I left the imaging center relieved and a little proud of myself for checking another thing off the mental to-do list.

Two days later, the phone rang.

They needed a follow-up scan. Nothing to worry about, they said—likely just a blurry image or a shadow that needed clarifying.

But curiosity got the best of me. I logged into the patient portal and opened the radiologist's report. It was a wall of unfamiliar medical language. I copied one of the long, technical terms and pasted it into Google. Article after article came up—clinical, dense, terrifying. One in particular stuck with me: the term almost always indicated malignancy.

My chest tightened. I called my parents and my brother, each of them with a background in medicine. That night, they were attending a hospital event, the kind my dad used to frequent before he retired. One of their oldest friends, the head of breast radiology, was there. They showed him the report.

He didn't sugarcoat it. "She needs a biopsy. Immediately."

But the earliest appointment in my area was a month away. There's no way my spiraling mind could wait a whole month for answers. That same doctor, our friend, told me to get on a plane. "Come home. We'll see you Monday morning."

The next afternoon, my brother showed up at my house—completely unannounced. He visited often, usually to spend time with us and play with our daughter, but never without giving us advance notice. This time was different.

He walked in quietly, and we sat together on the carpet. He looked up at me, eyes filled with tears. I had never seen him like that before—his face etched with a kind of sadness that words couldn't touch—a deep, aching sorrow.

My brother is the Medical Director of a Pediatric Intensive Care Unit. In my mind, it's the most challenging job in the world. He cares for children who are critically ill, many of them hovering between life and death. He's spent years delivering the kind of news no parent should ever hear, and somehow, he's always managed to carry both grace and grit—compassion balanced with the strength it takes to walk into the next room and try to save another life.

He's seen unimaginable things. But I had never seen *him* like this.

With a trembling voice, he told me he had sent my mammogram report to the head of radiology at his hospital—one of the top medical centers in the country. He said he knew the radiologist who read my scan personally. "He's one of the best," he told me. "He doesn't miss things."

Then he paused, searching for the right words. His voice dropped low.

"Let's just say it, I think you have cancer," he said gently. "I'm fairly confident."

The room felt still, heavy. My world had shifted in a sentence.

The next day, I flew back to my hometown.

I arrived at the breast center before the doors were even unlocked, my heart pounding louder than my footsteps, tears already running down my face. The waiting was unbearable. The uncertainty was heavier than any diagnosis could be.

The radiologist who performed my biopsy was a woman around my age, soft-spoken, deliberate. At one point, I asked her outright, "What do you think the results will be?"

She paused. "I think it's cancer."

Her voice was steady but kind.

I swallowed my fear and asked if there was any way to rush the results. She nodded and told me she understood—because she, too, was waiting for her own biopsy results. She'd had a procedure just the day before.

In that moment, something unspoken passed between us. Two mothers. Two women in limbo. We embraced—strangers, yet not strangers at all.

The next day, I was scheduled for a work trip in Los Angeles. I debated canceling it, but in the end, I went. I needed the distraction, the illusion of normalcy.

It was there, amidst back-to-back meetings, that I had my first flicker of light.

My colleague—someone I'd known for years—was driving us from one location to the next. I told her that I was waiting on results. She didn't flinch. Instead, she reached over, touched my hand, and said, "I had breast cancer twenty years ago. I've been cancer-free ever since."

Hope. Just a sliver. But enough.

That afternoon, while standing in the belly of Sofi Stadium during a meeting, my phone rang. I stepped away, heart racing.

It was our family friend, the radiologist.

He didn't hesitate.

"It's what we thought. It's cancer."

The world fell silent. Not quiet—silent. Like that movie scene where an explosion hits, and all you can hear is the ringing. I don't remember the rest of the meeting. I don't remember the drive to the hotel. It was all muffled under the weight of those two words.

I walked up to the front desk and asked to check out a day early. "I just got a call. I have cancer," I said flatly, barely recognizing my own voice. I wasn't looking for sympathy, just a refund on a night I wouldn't use. The woman behind the counter disappeared without a word.

Ten minutes later, she returned. "No problem," she said softly, and handed me a room key.

I rode the elevator in silence, and when I opened the door, I stopped cold.

She had moved me to the penthouse suite.

It was sprawling and beautiful—far too luxurious for what I was feeling. But I understood. It was her way of giving me something—anything—in the darkest hour of my life.

A moment of grace.

And in that moment, I let myself feel it. *The kindness of strangers.* The fragility of life. And the quiet strength that would carry me through what was coming next.

Finding Hope & Joy in Cancer

Chapter 2: When the World Stood Still

"In the middle of every difficulty lies opportunity." — Albert Einstein

If getting diagnosed with cancer was the moment the world screeched to a halt, then the years leading up to it were like the dramatic slow-motion montage before a car crash in a movie—chaotic, jam-packed, and weirdly poetic. Life had been full—love, work, a wedding (almost), a baby, a global pandemic—and I had been running on adrenaline and resilience. From the outside, life looked like a highlight reel. But beneath the surface, a chaotic cocktail of stress, sleepless nights, and self-neglect was brewing something entirely different. It was a cocktail only a tumor could love. Looking back, it's no mystery—those years were the perfect breeding ground. Cancer didn't come out of nowhere. It had been watching me skip workouts, stress over spreadsheets, and "power through" for years, probably rubbing its tiny cellular hands together, saying, "Soon."

The three years leading up to 2020 were a whirlwind of activity. I had started dating my best friend of 18 years—a love that had quietly grown in the background of my life like a rom-com waiting for its final scene. A year later, we were engaged, and I dove headfirst into planning my dream wedding. I used to joke that I would have become a wedding planner if only it didn't require working weekends —or managing the occasional fire-breathing bride. So this wedding—*our* wedding—became my passion project, and I loved every second of it.

We were set to get married on March 21, 2020, in a destination wedding in Mexico surrounded by our closest friends and family. It was everything I had dreamed of—sun, sand, love, laughter, and a weekend of celebration.

Then, just a week before the big day, everything began to unravel. The NCAA canceled its basketball tournament—one of the first seismic signs that COVID was more than just a whisper in the headlines. It was real. Each day brought worse news, and one by one, our guests began to call with apologies and concern. Six days before the wedding, it became heartbreakingly clear: we had to cancel.

The decision wasn't just about logistics—it was about responsibility. I couldn't bear the thought that someone might get sick because of us. What was supposed to be the happiest weekend of my life dissolved into a quiet kind of grief.

We knew we wanted to start a family, and it had always felt important to me to be married before trying to conceive. But time wasn't exactly on our side. I was nearing 40, and my soon-to-be husband was approaching 50. Two months later, we found the only place still marrying people in person—the DMV. Yes, the DMV. Not exactly the Pinterest wedding board I had envisioned.

A man at a desk typed a few things into his computer, and just like that, we were legally wed. No aisle, no music, no cake—just a government-issued receipt of romance.

My parents happened to be visiting my brother and me that weekend, so while we were out, they sprang into action. My mom stayed back at the house, cooking a celebration dinner, while my dad and brother— two grown men, both doctors—set off on a mission. They headed straight to Michaels and loaded up on poster board, puffy paint, glitter, and markers.

When we walked through the door, we were greeted by a bottle of champagne, a bouquet of roses, and a handmade sign that looked like it belonged at a kindergarten art fair—courtesy of two highly educated medical professionals. It was absolutely perfect.

Soon after, I began tracking my cycle. The tests never showed that I was ovulating, and I started to fear that maybe it was too late for me. At my annual exam, I braced for the word "menopause"—but instead, the doctor smiled gently and said, "You're pregnant."

Pregnant? I had only stopped taking birth control a month earlier and had been told it could take much longer. I wasn't ready. It was the Fourth of July, and we were surrounded by friends on our annual trip to Whitefish, Montana. I lied constantly about why I wasn't drinking— I wasn't ready to share. But just days later, at a follow-up appointment, the doctor told me my hormone levels weren't normal. I would likely miscarry within 24 to 48 hours.

It's hard to describe the feelings that came next—a mixture of loss and unexpected relief, which only made me feel guilty. I wasn't ready, but I had already begun to dream. The doctor advised me to wait a month to allow my body to reset. And during that time, something clicked: I realized I wasn't ovulating when I thought I was. My cycle was later than average. So, when the next month came, I knew exactly when it could happen—and this time, I was ready.

I told my husband I was pregnant before any test could confirm it. "How do you know?" he asked, amused. "I just do," I told him. I took tests every day, watching the second line grow darker with each passing moment. It was real. It was happening. And to me, it was nothing short of a miracle.

That first month, I walked every day, cradling my belly and singing softly: *It's you and me, baby. I dreamed of you. It's you and me, baby. My dream came true.*

A few weeks later, we visited my parents, and I surprised them with the news. I had set up my phone in the corner to record. My mom unwrapped a tiny onesie, looked at it, and suddenly screamed with joy, jumping up and down as if a baby were already inside. Her happiness was contagious—pure and unfiltered. Later that evening, I asked her to pray over my belly. Her words were soft and steady, and in that moment, I knew—somehow—we were going to be okay.

Thirty-eight weeks later, I gave birth to a beautiful baby girl.

A year earlier, as COVID shut down the world, I had accepted the role of COO and CMO of an early-stage wine company. I was a certified Level 2 sommelier—not something I had ever planned to use professionally, but I had a genuine passion for wine. This job, combining my love for wine with my background in business, was a dream. The founder was also a new mom and fully supported whatever maternity leave I needed.

But I never really took one.

I was still in my hospital bed, holding my hours-old daughter, when I found myself responding to work emails. I couldn't help myself. I didn't want to let go of the work I loved—or let anyone down.

Breastfeeding was its own mountain. My milk supply was low, and I found myself breastfeeding or pumping for 10–12 hours a day. When I finally started supplementing with formula, I felt like a failure. I knew how important breast milk was, and I felt crushed that I couldn't give our baby everything she needed. I cried almost every night—alone, in the dark, with a silent desperation no one saw.

For the first two months, our daughter needed to be held constantly. My husband and mom helped in every way they could, but there are some things only a mother can do. The exhaustion ran deep.

I remember, during my pregnancy, confidently telling friends that becoming a mom wouldn't slow me down. I'd still be up for trips, events, dinners—everything. One friend with grown children gently smiled and said, "Give it at least six weeks." I laughed it off, thinking, *Not me.*

Oh, how naïve I was.

Chapter 3: The Move, the Marriage, and the Middle of the Night

"There is no way to be a perfect mother, but a million ways to be a good one." — Jill Churchill

If there was one silver lining to the chaos of COVID, it was freedom—the freedom to work from anywhere, wear pajama pants 24/7, and order groceries without making awkward small talk. During my pregnancy, I craved warmth, sunshine, and the ability to walk outside without slipping on ice or dodging snow shovels. We chose Phoenix, Arizona, signed a six-month lease on a beautiful apartment, and settled into the desert heat just in time to welcome our daughter into the world. She was born at Shea Hospital in mid-April.

The timing couldn't have been better. When she was finally cleared to travel after her two-month vaccinations, we packed up and headed for Montana.

Correction: *I* packed up and moved.

Two months postpartum, and I packed every. Single. Box. Alone.

Why? Maybe it was the illusion of control. Maybe I needed to prove I could do it all. Maybe it was my misguided belief that asking for help meant I was failing. Most likely, it was all of the above with a sprinkle of hormonal delusion. Either way, I was determined to do it myself—because, clearly, sleep-deprived new moms are known for making rational decisions.

Montana was meant to be a pause—a place of rest, of help, of family. My husband and I looked forward to our first dinner date since becoming parents. Over dinner, I said what had been on my heart:

"We need to make sure we love each other first. We need to prioritize our relationship over our daughter."

He looked at me and said, "It's pretty hard not to love her more than everything else."

And just like that, something inside me cracked. Not shattered, but cracked—like when you drop a mug and it still holds coffee but feels a little more fragile.

I was sensitive. I'll own that. I was exhausted and insecure, and trying so hard to be everything to everyone. And in that moment, I felt like I had dropped down a few rungs—second, third, maybe even fourth place. Isn't that how people often say fathers feel when their wives prioritize the baby above all else? Turns out, the roles can just as easily be reversed.

We'd come to Montana to live with my parents for the summer. Both of us were working full-time, and finding childcare that felt safe and trustworthy in those early months was nearly impossible. My parents, especially my mom, stepped in with incredible love and care. I will always be grateful for that. In the quiet early mornings and in between Zoom calls, I watched as my mother held my daughter with the same tenderness she once gave me. It was beautiful and grounding.

As the world slowly began to reopen, it was time to head back to Colorado, where my husband's job was based. At the end of the year, we bought a house—my first house—and made the move.

I still wasn't comfortable putting our daughter in daycare. She was so young. So I found another family whose daughter was the same age. Together, we hired a nanny—warm, attentive, and loving, the kind of person you hope for when you leave your child in someone else's care. We alternated homes, and I got to watch the other little girl—so calm, so content, such an easy baby.

I was envious.

Our daughter never wanted to be still. She needed motion, engagement, presence—always. It was like parenting a hummingbird—a very cute, very busy hummingbird with a personal vendetta against sleep.

My husband's job kept him on the road. So, my days began early—up with the baby between 5 and 6 a.m., working as soon as the nanny arrived, and then back to full-time parenting the moment she left. Evenings were filled with bottles, baths, books, and bouncing. Once the baby was finally down, I'd either work more or clean the house. Then I'd collapse into bed, only to wake and do it all over again. Exhausted doesn't even begin to describe it.

On the outside, everything looked beautiful. I had the kind of career people envy—COO and CMO of a thriving startup, surrounded by smart, passionate people, building something exciting. *But inside, I was disappearing.* I hadn't seen a friend in over a year. All my free time was spent researching how to parent perfectly—sleep training, baby-led weaning, crawling, tummy time, motor skill development. I didn't just want to do it well; I wanted to do it perfectly. I wanted to do it flawlessly. Like a Type A mom of the year who also casually crushed board meetings.

Meanwhile, my husband parented on instinct. "This just feels right," he'd say. When the baby slept, so did he. I would quietly clean up, then round the corner to find him on the couch, watching golf—because nothing lulls you into a deep dad nap like the soothing tones of Jim Nantz and the gentle hum of a putting green. And slowly, quietly, resentment began to build—not just because I hadn't figured out how to ask for what I needed, but maybe also because he was channeling the energy of a golden retriever on a Sunday afternoon: sweet, loyal, and absolutely no help with the dishes.

His job was getting harder, the demands growing heavier, and we started fighting—all the time. The tension between us was constant, and I was miserable. But instead of talking about it, I held it all in. I didn't know how to say what I felt, so I said nothing at all. It sat inside me, dark and heavy, growing heavier by the day.

I wasn't angry at him. Okay—maybe a little. But mostly, I was angry at the pressure I put on myself. The impossible standards. The belief that love meant doing it all, flawlessly and without complaint. And slowly I realized that, eventually, something had to give.

Chapter 4: Surrender

"You only lose what you cling to." — Buddha.

Around our daughter's first birthday, I asked my husband a question I'd been holding in for months: *Are you happy?*

He paused and replied, "Not right now."

We had just argued—again. But I wasn't asking about the fight. I was asking about *us*. About everything.

It took everything I had to ask that question. Vulnerability doesn't come easily to me. I'm not a natural communicator. I grew up in a family that kept conflict behind closed doors. I never saw my parents fight, even though they did—no one modeled resolution—only avoidance. Conflict terrified me.

But a few years earlier, I met someone who would change the way I saw connection. She's now my best friend, and at the time, I was consulting for legendary sports agent Leigh Steinberg—our third time working together in my career. I invited her to the Super Bowl to help with all the chaos: media row, a 1,000+ person agency party, making sure NFL players got into the hottest events, and generally buzzing from task to task like a human Swiss Army knife with a never-ending to-do list.

I was running around making sure every last detail was flawless for a dinner with the executives, the veteran players, and their hot young quarterback, Patrick Mahomes. Yes, that Patrick Mahomes—before the MVPs and Super Bowl rings. And there I was, running a two-minute drill in heels, triple-checking menus, seating arrangements, and the décor I'd painstakingly designed over the past month, as if the entire NFL season hinged on whether the breadbasket showed up on time.

Later that weekend came one of my favorite "did that really happen?" moments. Patrick and his girlfriend (now wife), Brittany, showed up at the Maxim Magazine party. The security guard gave me that skeptical look that basically said, *Convince me.*

I leaned in: "He's going to be the starting quarterback for the Chiefs next season now that Alex Smith is gone."

The guy smirked. "You don't know that. I doubt it."

I wasn't about to debate NFL futures with a bouncer, so I pivoted: "He doesn't need to walk the red carpet, just let them in and have a good time." Thankfully, as Patrick and Brittany got closer, security relented. Crisis averted.

To this day, I wonder if that doorman tells his buddies over cocktails about how he almost turned away one of the greatest to ever play the game.

While I was busy managing every last detail, my friend noticed how tightly wound I was. I micromanaged everything, even the things she already had perfectly under control. Eventually, she turned to me and asked—kindly but directly—"Did I do something to upset you?"

It stopped me in my tracks. In my family, we often resorted to silence, retreat, or passive-aggressive comments when something was wrong. But her clarity, her kindness—it quietly tore down a wall I didn't even realize was there. Upon some self-reflection, I admitted that what had me wound so tightly wasn't just the chaos of the Super Bowl—it was my own insecurity. I wanted to appear perfect, the tireless, hardworking individual who never missed a beat. And beneath that, I didn't want to let down the man who had basically given me my PhD in sports business—Leigh Steinberg. I had started my career as his executive assistant, and a decade later, I wanted to prove that all his professional grooming had produced a capable and confident sports executive.

That simple moment with my friend led to one of the first truly honest and vulnerable conversations I'd ever had. And it showed me something I hadn't learned from any mentor, party, or press room: *real connection isn't built through perfection, but through communication.*

Still, I was far from fluent in that language. And in my marriage, I struggled to express what I needed or feared. I stuffed things down, hoping they'd just dissolve. But they never did.

Around that same time, a dear friend invited me to a healing ceremony. I'd never done one before, but several people I trusted swore by the life-changing insights it offered. I brought the idea to my husband, and he was open—even excited—to do it with me.

True to form, I entered the experience with a mental checklist: *What's my life's purpose? What should I do next? Am I on the right career path? Where should we live? How can I create a meaningful life for our daughter? How do I find a deeper connection—within myself, with others, with the world?*

I suppose I thought some divine voice would echo through the room and say, '*Amanda, here is your path. Follow it, and all will be well.*'

Before we began, we sat in a circle and shared our intentions. When I spoke mine—my long list of questions and hopes—the guide looked at me and said, "I hear a lot of doing. You want to *do*, to *fix*, to *plan*. But this experience is not about doing. It's about receiving. The more you try to control it, the less room you give the universe to speak."

His words didn't immediately sink in. I was raised on the principles of structure, goal-setting, and hard work. Every summer, my dad and I would set a goal for my golf game. One summer, the goal was simply to beat him on a single hole. If I did, I'd get a $100 bill. I achieved it, laminated that bill, and never spent it. The pride I felt was electric.

I carried that same energy into school. When I got a B+ in fourth grade, I swore I'd never get less than an A again—and I didn't. I became valedictorian. In college, after receiving a C on one of my first exams, I doubled down and studied 12 hours straight, day after day, to ensure it never happened again. One day, my parents called and said, "Are you sitting down?" I braced myself for bad news. Instead, they said, "We're worried you're not having enough *fun* in college." What parents say that?

I graduated at the top of my class—a semester early. My drive had always been my compass. So, when the guide asked me to let go of it, it felt like being told to release the only tool I knew how to use.

Still, I was all in.

The experience didn't give me the tidy list of answers I'd been hoping for. There was no booming voice from the heavens telling me where to live, what career to choose, or how to design a perfectly meaningful life for our daughter. Instead, it gave me something far more uncomfortable—and ultimately, more powerful.

It showed me just how tightly I was holding on. How hard I was trying to control, fix, and manage every moment of my life—right down to the way I was "supposed" to have a breakthrough. It made me confront the deep-rooted belief that my worth was tied to productivity. That if I wasn't achieving, I was falling behind.

But once I let go—once I stopped "doing" and simply allowed myself to "be"—I saw something I hadn't in a long time: joy. Pure, uncomplicated joy. I laughed. I felt light. I remembered what it felt like to play, to be present, to exist without constantly measuring the value of every second.

Of course, even in that joy, the old patterns crept in. I worried about ruining the experience for someone else. What if I was laughing too loudly? Was there a right way to enjoy this? Classic overachiever move—grading myself on how well I was letting go.

Physically, I wasn't in great shape either. My back had gone out the day before (perfect timing), and I needed rest more than revelation. But that space gave me time to reconnect with my husband in a way we hadn't in ages. We talked—not just about logistics, diapers, and what was for dinner, but about us. About who we wanted to be, as individuals and as partners.

I came away with fewer answers than I'd expected—but far more clarity. *The experience taught me to block time for stillness. To receive. To stop constantly striving and start simply being.*

And maybe, just maybe, it didn't just shift something inside me.

It brought us back to each other.

It was summertime, and for a while, everything felt perfectly aligned. Life had found its rhythm. My husband had just closed out the fiscal year as one of the top sales performers at his company—a huge win. That success gave him the leverage to ask for a new territory, one that would finally bring us back to Arizona. It was something we had both been hoping for. The company agreed, and we started planning our move for the winter. It felt like the start of a new chapter.

Professionally, I had found fresh inspiration consulting for a real estate development start-up. The work focused on preparing materials for a capital raise of over $1 billion, and since it was project-based, I could take it on during nights and weekends. I still loved my full-time role as COO and CMO of the wine company—the team, the product, the mission—but I was craving more. More challenge. More upside. More purpose.

With the same conviction we brought to the wine business, we also decided to make a significant personal financial investment in the real estate development company. We were all-in—energized, ambitious, on fire with possibility. The future felt wide open.

Two weeks later, the phone rang. It was the mammogram imaging center.

And everything changed.

Chapter 5: Upload

"Owning our story and loving ourselves through that process is the bravest thing we'll ever do." — Brené Brown

After returning home from my work trip in Los Angeles, the world turned dark. Not just emotionally—it felt physically darker, heavier. I didn't even know where to begin.

I called my OB/GYN, hoping for some direction, a next step, a sense of structure. Their response: "I guess, try to find a breast cancer surgeon?"

It landed like a thud. Uncertainty wrapped in indifference. I hung up thinking, Wow, glad we cleared that up. Should I also Google how to rebuild an engine while I'm at it?

My parents, trying to help in the way only loving and slightly panicked parents can, reached out to a close friend—an oncologist. He wasn't a breast cancer specialist, but at least he could walk us through the biopsy report without using Google Translate for medical speak. He confirmed what I already suspected: yes, I would need treatment. Yes, I would need surgery. It wasn't a question of *if,* but *how soon.*

The only other frame of reference I had for breast cancer was my best friend from college. She was diagnosed in her late twenties. I held her hand in the hospital after her double mastectomy and helped care for her in the days that followed. She went through it all—chemo, radiation, every grueling step. Years later, the cancer came back. It spread. And eventually, it took her life.

That was one of my only data points. *Breast cancer meant death.*

I could barely breathe when I looked at my daughter—just 18 months old—and thought, *What have I done?* How selfish was I to bring a child into the world only to leave her so soon? I became consumed with the fear that I had doomed her to grow up motherless. I made my husband promise—*no matter what happens*, he would live close to my family. That he'd let my parents and brother help raise her. She needed to know where she came from.

I didn't even have a treatment plan yet. But my brain leapt straight to the worst-case scenario. If catastrophizing were an Olympic sport, I'd have taken gold. I couldn't stop myself.

In the days that followed, I buried myself in work. I put on a smile, hit every meeting, answered every email, and pretended—flawlessly—that everything was fine. You'd have thought I was gunning for "Employee of the Month While Secretly Falling Apart." But the minute the workday ended and the mask came off, I crumbled. I cried in the shower. I cried in the dark. I cried silently while folding laundry. My grief was anticipatory, imagined—but still, it was real.

And yet, I'm a doer. A problem-solver. A spreadsheet-loving, solution-seeking, give-me-a-plan-and-I'll-execute-the-hell-out-of-it kind of person. If there was a way to survive this, I was going to find it.

The first step was telling people. I needed support—but the idea of dozens of one-on-one conversations, each ending in tears, was too much. I couldn't get through even a sentence without breaking down. And I knew everyone would ask the same questions: *What happened? What's next? Are you okay?*

I asked my husband, "Would it be weird if I just recorded a video? Sent it to our closest people and then maybe posted it on social media?"

He looked at me with soft eyes and said, "Do whatever makes it easiest for you."

So I did.

I sat in front of my phone and pressed the record button. Three minutes. Raw. Gut-wrenching. Honest. I spoke through tears. My voice cracked. I said the words out loud that I had barely let settle in my mind: *I have cancer.*

Then I hit upload.

And just like that, I told the world.

Chapter 6: The Shift

"You get in life what you have the courage to ask for." — Oprah Winfrey

About six months before my diagnosis—right after the not-so-casual life-reset ceremony—I started working with an executive well-being coach. Looking back, I realize how much I owe her. She didn't just help me become a better leader and find clarity in my work. She helped me create a more peaceful home, a more intentional life—and maybe even stopped me from turning into a full-time tornado of stress. Honestly, she was nothing short of magic.

Our November session happened over Zoom, just days after my world had unraveled. The moment my camera turned on, she leaned in with that signature psychic-like stare, eyes soft but sharp, and asked, "What's wrong? What's going on?"

She hadn't even said hello, yet somehow already knew.
What I didn't know then was that she had walked alongside many executive women through their cancer journeys. And right there, on that call, she gave me a piece of advice I'll never forget—advice that became my anchor:

Be direct.

Tell people exactly what you need—and what you don't. Be clear about what's helpful and what's not. Don't leave them guessing. Don't pretend you're fine. Ask for what you actually want.

It seems simple now, but at the time, it felt revolutionary. I'd spent my life dancing around discomfort, sugarcoating hard truths, and cushioning everyone else's feelings like I was auditioning for emotional Cirque du Soleil.

But now? I didn't have the energy to juggle anyone else's expectations. I barely had the strength to hold my own fear.

So, I took her advice, and when it came time to share my story publicly, that's exactly what I did.

I recorded that three-minute video—raw, honest, filmed in one take with no script and very puffy eyes. And I told the truth:

How am I doing? Not great. When I first found out, I fell into a deep black hole—not for me, but for my daughter. I kept thinking about her growing up without a mother and how that would shape her life...

What I really need right now is your prayers and your good thoughts—every single one you can send my way and to our family...

If you know any stories about people who've beaten cancer—who are cancer-free for five, ten, fifteen, twenty years—I want them. I need those stories.

And I'll take any good news. I'm trying to smile. I'm trying to stay positive. So, send me your good news, your funny stories—anything that brings light. I need it.

I also want to say thank you in advance for every message. I promise I'm reading them all, even if I don't have the energy to respond. Please don't take it personally if I don't reply. Just know that I love you—and I appreciate you.

What happened next was overwhelming. The floodgates opened. Support poured in from people I hadn't heard from in years—old friends, former colleagues, even that girl I sat next to in junior year chemistry who once lent me a pencil and apparently still cared deeply.

🩶 You will be the strongest mommy after you beat this battle!

Sending you all the love and positive thoughts Mandy—You are one of the strongest and most inspiring women I know, and I know you got this 🩶🩶🩶

Sending you and your family so much strength, love and light, Amanda! 🩶

You are a beacon of light, thanks for your strength and vulnerability to share this here. We love you and are here for you however we can be!

Sending So much love and strength your way beautiful friend! We love you and you're not fighting alone. I know you can kick cancers ass! 💪🦾✨🩶

The outpouring was humbling. It was also deeply affirming, encouraging, and comforting. I wasn't alone.

But alongside all that love, there were also the moments I needed someone to cut through the cheerleading with raw honesty. Later that week, I went on a walk with my brother and admitted that I knew I *should* have a positive attitude, but I couldn't shake the dark cloud of despair hanging over me. He looked at me and said, "Sister, I hear you and you're right, but give yourself some grace to feel all the hard feelings. This is just shitty. I'm sorry you're having to go through this." I didn't even realize how much I needed to hear that until he said it out loud—that blunt truth that, yes, I'd been dealt a really crap hand. It gave me permission to stop pretending I was fine and feel what I felt.

And in that wave of kindness and truth came two life-changing gifts— recommendations from friends I deeply respected, all from completely different corners of my life.

One told me to read *The Obstacle Is the Way* by Ryan Holiday. The other sent me a link to an interview between Jay Shetty and Dr. Joe Dispenza.

At the time, I didn't realize it, but those two suggestions would quietly shift the course of my entire journey—just as much as the diagnosis itself.

Chapter 7: The Obstacle Becomes the Way

"Sometimes the very walls that block us are the ones that teach us how to climb."
— Unknown

Two weeks after my diagnosis—when I was barely eating, barely sleeping, and completely unraveling—I'd wake up every morning at 4 a.m., begging—*please let this be a bad dream.* And when it wasn't, the fear would grip me all over again like a surprise party I never wanted.

I boarded a flight with a desperate hope for escape, or at least distraction. I had downloaded *The Obstacle Is the Way* by Ryan Holiday after a friend I deeply respected insisted that I read it. I had no idea it would become my first tether back to hope.

I sat in my cramped airplane seat, noise-canceling headphones on, trying not to ugly-cry into my Biscoff cookies. As I listened, it felt like every word had been written directly for me.

The book isn't about cancer, or illness, or even personal tragedy. It's about ancient Stoic philosophy—and how we, as humans, often can't control what happens to us, but we always have control over how we respond.

That book became my first lifeline. It cracked open a new way of thinking. What if this diagnosis—this terrifying, unwanted thing—wasn't just something to survive? What if it were the thing that would change everything? The thing that would finally set my life on the path it was always meant to follow?

One of the first lessons that hit me was this:

"The obstacle in the path becomes the path. Never forget, within every obstacle is an opportunity to improve our condition."

I'd spent weeks drowning in fear, replaying worst-case scenarios, bargaining with fate. I kept asking *Why is this happening to me?* But the question I needed to be asking was *What is cancer here to teach me?*

Another idea that lodged itself into my brain: perception. How we see a situation often matters more than the situation itself. Holiday writes that if you can train yourself to see obstacles as opportunities, you stop being a passive victim of your circumstances. You take your power back. And I thought, '*Yes, please.' I'll take two.*

I started to ask myself:

What if this diagnosis wasn't a death sentence, but a wake-up call?
What if it forced me to slow down, reevaluate, and finally put my health first?
What if it became the catalyst for living with more purpose, more clarity, more presence?

I also learned about action—the discipline of turning fear into forward motion. The idea isn't to bulldoze your way through life, but to take intentional steps, no matter how small, even when you're afraid, especially when you're afraid.

So, I stopped letting fear paralyze me. I started making lists. I booked doctor appointments. I asked questions. I educated myself. I prepared for battle—not with cancer, but with my own spiraling thoughts.

And finally, the most humbling lesson: the discipline of will. Understanding that we won't always win, but we can always choose how we face the hard stuff. Courage. Dignity. Resilience. Even if we're wearing mismatched socks and haven't washed our hair in four days.

By the time the plane landed, something inside me had shifted. I wasn't magically healed. I wasn't even hopeful yet. But I felt... steadier. Stronger. Like maybe I wasn't powerless after all.

I realized then—and I believe it still—
The obstacle doesn't block the path. It becomes the path.

This was my path now. And I was ready to walk it.

From that moment on, a question began to take root in my mind, one I couldn't shake:

What is this teaching me?

And more importantly—

How can I use it to make my world, and the world, better?

Chapter 8: Choosing My Team

"If you want to go fast, go alone. If you want to go far, go together." — African Proverb

After a week of spinning in emotional circles, philosophical reckonings, and ceremony-induced self-reflection, I landed squarely in logistics mode. I had officially entered my Type A comeback era. It was time to *do* something.

With my husband traveling most weekdays for work, and a wild, curious 18-month-old who had the energy of a caffeinated squirrel, we made the call: we'd temporarily relocate to Southern California to be near my parents. Trading snow for sunshine while tackling a cancer diagnosis? Not exactly a hard sell. It felt like an unexpected silver lining in a season that felt otherwise stormy.

The move brought a strange kind of comfort—but also a new wave of anxiety. Moving meant starting over with my medical care.

I did what any modern woman facing a life-altering diagnosis does—I turned to Google.

Big mistake.

Within minutes, I was drowning in "Top 10 Cancer Centers," celebrity oncologist profiles, survival statistics, Reddit rabbit holes, and a seemingly endless scroll of doom. I felt like I was trying to assemble a life raft from WebMD and Yelp reviews.

So, I did what any panicked, overwhelmed, slightly spiraling adult would do: I phoned a friend.

I called one of my closest childhood friends whose mom had been a nurse in the area for decades. I thought that if anyone had a backstage pass to the medical elite, it would be her.

"I don't," she admitted. "But one of my friends trained with a top breast surgeon at USC. I'll text her now."

I wish I could say the rest happened *just like that*. But it didn't.

It took countless hours.
Dozens of phone calls with administrators.
Repeated imaging tests.
An act of God to get my medical records to land in the right hands.
Begging various medical offices to accept faxes, as if it were 1996 (which they didn't).
Meticulous calendar juggling to make it all happen before the holidays.

After enough back-and-forth to rival a season of "Survivor: Insurance Edition," I landed consultations at two leading institutions: USC Keck Medical Center and City of Hope. I didn't want one opinion. I wanted a full-on medical consensus.

Finally, a week later, I walked into USC Keck Medical Center with my mom by my side.

My mom—calm, collected, a quiet force—was the ideal companion. She took detailed notes, asked smart questions, and sat with me through every uncomfortable pause. But more than anything, she brought the steady kind of love only a mom can offer on a day like that.

At USC, we met the full roster in one go—like being introduced to the starting lineup before the big game: the breast surgeon, the medical oncologist, and the support staff. They walked me through everything, point by point, until I could practically see the playbook in my head. For the first time since my diagnosis, I felt less like a case number and more like a person they actually knew.

The verdict: I had triple-positive breast cancer—estrogen receptor positive (ER+), progesterone receptor positive (PR+), and HER2 positive.

Not the worst-case scenario, but far from the easiest path. It wasn't the slow-moving, "watch and wait" kind either.

Triple-positive came with both good news and hard news.

The good? It tends to respond well to treatment. There are effective targeted therapies designed for this exact combination.

The hard? Treatment would be long. Grueling. And I'd have decisions to make at every turn.

Here was the plan they laid out:

- Six rounds of chemotherapy, given every three weeks over four months.
- A combination of targeted immunotherapy drugs—Herceptin and Perjeta— administered alongside chemo.
- After chemo, surgery. My choice: lumpectomy with radiation, single mastectomy, or double mastectomy. The outcomes, they said, were statistically similar in terms of recurrence. The decision would be personal. (No pressure.)
- Post-surgery, depending on what they found, I might need Kadcyla—a powerful targeted therapy—for 14 more rounds. If no residual disease showed up, I'd continue with maintenance Herceptin and Perjeta.

I nodded, took notes, and internally screamed. But okay—we had a plan.

The next stop was City of Hope.

The process there had a different rhythm—more like walking into a major airport on a busy travel day. Lots of people, a steady hum of activity, and a few moments where I wasn't totally sure which line I was supposed to be in. But the doctor?

A literal beam of light in a white coat.

She was warm, positive, and somehow made me believe I could do this—even though she was essentially calling the same plays as the USC team. Her presence alone felt like therapy.

I didn't leave with a clearer logistics plan, but I left with something harder to measure and just as important: HOPE.

And in that moment, I realized something—plans are great, but sometimes what you really need is a coach who makes you believe you can win.

On the two-hour drive back to my parents' house, the emotional dam broke.

I'd kept my businesslike mask on all day—asking questions, taking notes, staying stoic. But the moment we got in the car, it cracked wide open. I collapsed in tears.

How was I supposed to choose? This wasn't like picking a dentist or deciding between two wedding venues. This was my *life*.

That night, I tossed and turned. I stared at the ceiling and imagined every outcome. By morning, though, the clarity had come—gently, but firmly.

City of Hope had been exactly what I needed to hear—a reminder that this didn't have to be the end of my story. That I could—and would—get through this.

But when it came to care, I knew in my gut:
USC was my team.

They had the systems, the structure, the collaborative care model—and for my Type A, overachiever brain, that was like a weighted blanket of comfort. I wanted the *full* playbook, color-coded tabs, and maybe even a pop quiz to make sure everyone studied. If there was a gold-star version of cancer care, I was signing up.

And here's the kicker: I'm a Notre Dame alum. Choosing USC felt a little like asking your archrival to walk you down the aisle. But when your life's on the line, even Touchdown Jesus would understand—sometimes you root for the Trojans.

I could hold both: hope *and* precision. Spirit *and* science.

And finally—after weeks of questions, chaos, and consultation—I had my team.

And now, I had a plan.

Chapter 9: Becoming My Own Healer

"The wound is the place where the Light enters you." — Rumi

By the time chemo was scheduled, I was still determined to live—not just survive, not just get through it, but actually *live* through it. If cancer was going to crash the party, it was going to have to work around my calendar. I asked my oncologist if we could schedule treatments around the holidays—and, more critically, our long-awaited family trip to Hawaii in January.

To my surprise, we managed to make it work. Maybe the cancer was feeling generous.

Exactly five weeks after I got the call confirming my diagnosis—and two and a half weeks after a blur of consults, scans, and portal logins—I had my port placement and my first infusion scheduled. There was a plan. A path. A start line.

Ironically, it was in that waiting period—the space between knowing what I faced and actually starting treatment—that I felt a strange sense of calm. The storm of uncertainty had been the worst part. With a plan in place, I found myself breathing again. The fog hadn't cleared, but I could finally see a few feet ahead.

Even when a second biopsy revealed a second tumor in the same breast—a blow that might have shattered me weeks earlier—I didn't spiral. If anything, it brought clarity. I'd been agonizing over whether to do a lumpectomy or mastectomy. The decision was now made for me. Lumpectomy was off the table. I'd have a double mastectomy.

The obstacle is the way, I reminded myself—again.

It was around this time that I turned to the second life-changing recommendation I had received: the work of Dr. Joe Dispenza.

But it wasn't the science alone that hooked me—it was an interview. Jay Shetty, with his calm voice, warm energy, and genuinely curious questions, interviewed Dr. Joe in a way that felt less like a podcast and more like an intervention tailored just for me. Jay brought such presence and depth to the conversation that I found myself leaning in, rewinding, and taking notes. Not because I had to, but because it was the first time since my diagnosis that something made me feel powerful again.

Jay had this gentle way of peeling back the layers—asking the questions I didn't even realize I needed answered. And Dr. Joe delivered. He teaches that our thoughts create our reality—not in a fluffy, motivational way, but grounded in neuroscience and quantum physics. His research centers on how the brain and body interact—and how, through meditation and intentional thought, we can literally rewire our neural pathways, shift our emotional patterns, and even influence our physical health.

Dr. Joe teaches that we're not defined by our past, our DNA, or our diagnosis. We are defined by the thoughts we rehearse, the emotions we live in, and the future we choose to imagine. At first, I was skeptical. Was this just spiritual self-help with a sprinkle of science? But the more I listened, the more I realized this wasn't about escaping reality—it was about engaging with it differently. Could changing your thoughts really change your life… or your body?

His core message hit me right where I was standing:
We are not prisoners of our circumstances.
We are not defined by our diagnosis.
And we have more power over our health—and our future—than we've been taught to believe.

His concept of "living in the end" hit me like a lightning bolt. Instead of waking up every morning consumed by fear or worst-case scenarios, Dr. Joe teaches you to visualize the outcome you desire—and live as though it's already true. To feel, with every cell in your body, what it would be like to be healthy, whole, vibrant, and free. Live it—every day.

So, I started practicing.

Every single day, I would close my eyes and see myself healed. I would picture myself playing on the beach with my daughter, laughing, running, cancer-free.

I would imagine walking into my oncologist's office to hear the words, "There's no evidence of disease." I would feel joy—not forced positivity, but real, embodied JOY—and let it settle deep in my heart.

I learned that by doing this consistently, I wasn't just "thinking happy thoughts." I was literally training my body to experience a future reality before it happened. I was turning hope into a practice.

And it wasn't just about healing my body.

Dr. Joe's work taught me how often I lived in reaction—reacting to fear, to pressure, to other people's expectations. He taught me that if I stayed in those old patterns, I'd keep recreating the same emotional reality over and over again.

Through his meditations, I learned how to sit with myself—sometimes for hours—breathing, visualizing, surrendering. I stopped chasing certainty and started practicing presence. Gratitude became my medicine. Stillness became my sanctuary.

I realized I didn't want to just survive cancer. I wanted this experience to transform me.

So I made a quiet commitment to myself:
This wasn't going to be a chapter I endured.
This was going to be the beginning of my real life.

And slowly, I began to feel... different.

I felt calmer.

I felt lighter.
I felt like I wasn't just waiting for the chemo to save me.

I was saving myself, one thought at a time.

Looking back, I believe this shift—this choice to take responsibility for my inner world—was the real beginning of my healing.

Not just from cancer. This was about healing from years—maybe decades—of control, perfectionism, and fear. I was shedding old stories, outdated identities, and the belief that life only happened *to* me.

Now, I was letting life move *through* me.

Cancer would take its toll on my body, yes. But it would also give me back my life in a way nothing else ever could. A clearer path. A deeper truth. A second chance at living a life that actually felt like mine.

This was the remarkable transformation I never saw coming.

Chapter 10: A Peaceful Heart

"When you forgive, you don't change the past—you change your future."
— Unknown

Cancer taught me quickly that I couldn't carry old grudges and new battles at the same time. If I wanted strength for treatment, I had to lay down the weight of resentment and pick up peace instead. Making amends—whether with others or with myself—became less about fixing the past and more about freeing my heart for the fight ahead.

It took every ounce of courage—because let's be honest, confrontation ranks right up there with dental work and swimsuit shopping on my "least favorite activities" list—but I did it. I had some "loose ends" that needed tying, and cancer had a way of whispering, *"Do it now, don't wait."*

One was with a lifelong friend. Things had gone sideways, and instead of picking up the phone, I played it safe and recruited a mutual friend to play Switzerland and set up a play date. The truth was, decades of friendship were tangled up in a big ball of misunderstanding, and it hurt to be at odds with someone who had been such a constant in my life. But the minute we sat down and had a real heart-to-heart, it was like no time had passed at all. Just like that—back to besties.

The other situation was a business deal that had left me stewing. So, I did what any woman in cancer treatment might do: I put on my big-girl pants and sent a message that basically said, "I'm going through cancer treatment and I want to clear the air." (Pro tip: dropping the big "C" card tends to get a quick and heartfelt reply.) We ended up having an honest conversation where I learned he had truly believed his actions were fair, even if they hadn't felt that way to me. By the end, the frustration melted into understanding, and we shared what I can only describe as a giant virtual bear hug.

Finding Hope & Joy in Cancer

Here's what I learned in the process: peace doesn't come gift-wrapped, delivered to your doorstep like an Amazon package. You have to go out, face the awkward, and sometimes swallow a bit of pride. Making amends wasn't about keeping score or proving who was right—it was about lightening the load I was carrying into treatment. When you're staring down chemo chairs, scan results, and the very real possibility that life might not look the same again, suddenly that old grudge you've been clinging to loses its shine.

The funny thing is, the people I reached out to weren't walking around feeling weighed down like I was. They had moved on with their lives. I was the one still lugging around the baggage. And once I set it down, I realized just how much space it had been taking up in my heart.

Did every attempt end in a Hallmark moment? For me, surprisingly, yes—and I'll always be grateful for that. But here's the thing: not every attempt will end that way, and that's okay. Some people may not be ready to meet you halfway, and you can't control that. What you *can* control is showing up with honesty and kindness. Even if the response isn't what you hoped for, simply saying your piece and letting go can bring its own kind of peace. And that's the gift: knowing you've done your part.

Cancer demanded enough of my energy—I wasn't going to let bitterness or regret siphon off any more. By making amends where I could, I cleared the clutter in my heart and made room for hope, laughter, and the kind of joy that actually *fuels* healing. And I can tell you: a peaceful heart is a powerful ally in the chemo chair.

I learned that making amends isn't about fixing the past; it's about freeing your heart so you have room for hope.

Chapter 11: The Unexpected Counseling

"Love does not consist in gazing at each other, but in looking outward together in the same direction." — Antoine de Saint-Exupéry

When I scheduled my second opinion at City of Hope, I expected cutting-edge medicine, brilliant doctors, and maybe a few new questions to ask my team at USC. What I didn't expect was a mandatory couples counseling session.

Yes—*mandatory.*

At first, it caught me off guard. We weren't exactly on the verge of divorce—I mean, we were barely arguing. We were just two overtired parents clinging to a toddler's nap schedule and our shared survival instincts. But when City of Hope said every couple had to meet with a licensed therapist before starting treatment, I didn't push back. Honestly, I was intrigued. If there was bonus wisdom to collect—something that might help us get ahead of the emotional tidal wave—I was all in. After all, I was already juggling scans, surgery consults, and scheduling chemo around a trip to Hawaii. Why not add marriage prep to the mix?

So, there we were: sitting in my home office, side by side in front of the computer, waiting for a stranger to diagnose the state of our marriage over Zoom. The counselor greeted us with a warm smile and the kind of calm demeanor that instantly disarmed both of us.

"Before we talk about treatment," she said gently, "we need to talk about your team—you two. Because how you navigate this together will impact everything."

Honestly? She wasn't wrong.

I don't remember every word, but a few insights from that session wedged themselves into our bones. They became the emotional infrastructure we didn't know we needed.

Lesson 1: You're Both on Different Journeys—and That's Okay.

The counselor explained that while I would be the one going through chemotherapy, surgery, and all the physical effects of cancer, my husband would be on his own parallel journey—one of fear, helplessness, and watching someone he loves suffer.

"It will feel different for each of you," she said. "And you'll each cope in your own way."

That hit me harder than I expected. I had been so focused on *my* pain, *my* fear, *my* treatment, that I hadn't even considered the weight my husband was carrying. The helplessness of standing by, wanting to fix it—and knowing he couldn't.

It gave me a new lens of empathy. And it gave him permission to feel his own grief without guilt.

Lesson 2: Communicate the Hard Stuff—Even When It's Ugly.

"We see too many couples fall apart because they don't talk about the hard things," she said. "You have to speak the fear. Name the resentment. Say the thing you're afraid to say—before it grows into something bigger."

Oofta.

Cue the highlight reel of every moment I'd swallowed my stress, smiled through pain, or braved the day when all I wanted was to collapse. My default setting had always been: Be strong. Don't rock the boat. Keep going.

But that didn't work here.

This was our wake-up call. Cancer wasn't just a physical battle. It was going to test every corner of our relationship—and the only way through was together, with raw, honest communication.

That challenge stuck with me. And it showed up in ways I never expected.

I remember one fight—not even what it was about—but I'll never forget how it ended. My old instinct would have been to hold my ground until I "won" or walk away altogether. But that time, I stopped mid-argument, looked him in the eyes, and said:

"I need you to be better than me."

It wasn't a jab. It was me admitting I didn't have it in me to fight. I needed him to rise above, because I couldn't.

He immediately started laughing—a genuine, heartfelt laugh—and pulled me into a hug.

"Ok," he said with a smile. "I can try to do that."

That moment became a turning point. It broke the tension in the best possible way. And from that point on, we rarely fought again throughout my treatment. We had found a new rhythm—a grace neither of us had before. And we learned that sometimes, the most loving thing you can do is wave a little white flag and ask your person to take the lead.

Lesson 3: Define Your Roles—Before the Crisis Hits.

The counselor encouraged us to talk openly about what support would look like. Did I want him at every appointment? Did I need space after treatment days? How would we handle household responsibilities, childcare, and work during the hardest weeks?

It sounds simple. But defining those roles before we were in the thick of it saved us from so many potential blow-ups down the road.

We agreed:

- My mom would be at every chemo infusion and every major appointment. He would stay home and take care of our daughter with my dad.
- I would ask for—not expect—help when I needed it.
- We would lean on family when we needed it with our daughter.
- And above all, we would check in with each other regularly— not just about logistics, but about how we were *really* doing.

It wasn't about rigid rules. It was about knowing who was driving which part of the bus—and when to switch seats.

Lesson 4: You're a Team. And Teams Win Together or Lose Together.

"We know that couples who see themselves as a team—not just patient and caregiver—tend to weather this storm better," she said. "It's not about keeping score. It's about having each other's backs."

That simple statement reframed everything.

It wasn't about who was sacrificing more. It wasn't about tallying up who was more exhausted. It wasn't about blaming each other when stress boiled over.

We were on the same side of the battle.

When we ended that session, I felt like we had been handed a quiet but powerful set of tools—ones we didn't even know we were missing, and it gave us the grace to use them when it mattered most.

When the darkest days came, we leaned on each other instead of pulling away.

We chose to be a team.
We chose to speak the hard things.
We chose to give each other the space—and the grace—we both needed.

That unexpected session at City of Hope didn't just prepare us for cancer, it gave us a map.

And sometimes, all you need is a map to find your way through the wilderness together.

And as it turns out, the best way to get through the hard stuff?

Book the counseling session before things get hard. Even if you think you don't need it. *Especially* if you think you don't need it.

Chapter 12: Day One – Port, Poison, and Presence

"Courage is not the absence of fear, but the triumph over it." — Nelson Mandela

The day had arrived—my first chemotherapy treatment *and* port placement. A double-header. A duathlon of surrender and strength. I'd like to say I floated into it full of wisdom and Zen-like calm, but let's be real: I had one foot in warrior mode and one foot nervously googling "what snacks make chemo suck less."

Mentally, I was as ready as one can be when voluntarily signing up to be pumped full of poison. I had visualized calm. I had prepped my body. My bags were packed with healthy snacks, a heated blanket, headphones, and a playlist full of gentle voices telling me I was the universe. My mom and I drove to L.A. the night before to avoid traffic, booked a hotel near USC Keck, and tried to treat it like we were in town for a spa day. Spoiler: It was not that.

When I arrived at USC Keck Hospital, I was ushered into the pre-op room to get ready for the port placement procedure. A port, for those unfamiliar, is a small medical device surgically inserted beneath the skin—typically in the chest—with a catheter that leads to a major vein. It lets the chemo go straight into your bloodstream without needing a new IV every visit. Basically, it's VIP access for your veins.

The doctor who would be performing the procedure came in to introduce himself. He had that seasoned, silver-haired, and calm energy look that immediately put me at ease. He kindly explained the process and handed me his phone to sign the digital consent form. And that's when I noticed it—his hand was trembling.

Trembling.

This man was about to place a catheter into my heart-adjacent vein, and his hand looked like it belonged to someone trying to hold a cup of coffee during an earthquake.

I froze. My internal voice was screaming: *Wait, what? Is this safe? Is this really happening?*

But then something shifted in me. I closed my eyes. Took a deep breath. A full, cleansing inhale. I reminded myself: *You are safe. This man has done this a thousand times. Tremors happen. You've got this. Trust.*

And he *did* have it. When the port was removed nearly two years later, multiple nurses complimented on how beautifully it had been placed. Like, Michelangelo-level vein access. Hand tremor? Irrelevant. My panic? Temporary. The port? A masterpiece.

During the procedure itself, I stayed chatty—I asked the doctor about his family, we laughed about something funny I don't remember, it's all a pleasant blur. I even remember commenting—through the fog of sedation—on a stranger's beautiful boots in the recovery area. I told her they were "fabulous" and gave her a thumbs-up. I was high on love, hope, and sedation meds.

That's when I recorded a short, hilarious video and posted it on social media. I don't remember exactly what I said, but apparently, I was enthusiastic, loopy, and very, very sincere. Friends and family messaged me all day with encouragement—and plenty of laughing emojis.

But once I was wheeled into the chemo infusion center, the tone shifted. The nurses were kind but direct. They explained everything in excruciating detail—how each drug would work, the potential reactions, and what to look out for. They had an almost militaristic readiness, monitoring me like a hawk for every sign of an allergic response or sudden drop in blood pressure.

I received four agents that day:

Herceptin and Perjeta, targeted therapies designed to fight my specific HER2+ cancer cells.

Taxol and Carboplatin, two of the heavy hitters in the chemo world—known for their effectiveness, but also for their brutal side effects (chemo powerhouses with the charm of a chainsaw).

The infusion took hours longer than I expected. I was given pre-meds, saline flushes, and an infusion schedule that made international air travel look casual.

At one point, they gave me Benadryl to prevent allergic reactions, and I fell into a deep, dreamless sleep. It was the first true rest I'd had in days.

We stayed overnight in the hotel again, and surprisingly, the next morning, I felt... not awful. We went for a short walk, and I only got dizzy near the end. I remember feeling cautiously optimistic. We ate a beautiful salad on the patio back home, and I thought, *Hey... maybe this chemo thing won't be so bad after all.*

Cue the dramatic irony.

Later, the tsunami hit.

By nightfall, the side effects descended like a dark, rolling fog. The nausea, the bone pain, the mouth sores, the chills, the constipation, the diarrhea. (Yes, both. It defies logic.) My skin burned. My taste buds ghosted me. I felt like I had aged 40 years overnight. I'd read about the side effects. The nurses had warned me. But nothing prepares you for the moment your body becomes unrecognizable to you.

I won't go into every detail here—Google "chemo side effects" and check all the boxes. That was my week—a slow, disorienting descent into physical misery. I needed help with everything. I even had a full-blown panic attack. Not because of the pain—but because I realized there was no escape from my body. No exit ramp. Just the long, uphill climb through it all.

But I also found a tiny sliver of escape—and eventually, power—in a most unexpected place.

Meditation.

Every time I closed my eyes and put on a guided practice, I could feel myself leave my body. I floated above the pain. My chest softened. My gut settled. For those 30 or 60 minutes—sometimes longer—I didn't feel sick. I felt *nothing*. And then afterward, for a while, I still felt lighter. Like my body had remembered what it was like to be okay.

I was meditating daily—sometimes twice a day—and it became my sacred space. My sanctuary. The one thing that gave me back a sense of control.

That's when I decided to take Dr. Joe Dispenza's full online course.

I'd already been practicing his meditations for a few weeks. But I wanted to understand the science behind what I was feeling. I wanted to know why meditation worked—not just how. And more than anything, I wanted to learn how to use the power of my mind to heal, to visualize, to stay alive.

Lying in bed, body aching and vision blurred, I clicked through lesson after lesson. I learned about neuroplasticity, energy fields, quantum intention, and how thought alone can alter biology. It sounds lofty—and at times, unbelievable—but it *was* believable to me, because I was living it.

Before cancer, I was terrible at self-care. I poured myself into others, as if it were my full-time job—minus the benefits. I ran myself ragged and thought 'rest' was just a fancy word for laziness. I took pride in doing more than I should and treating burnout like a personality trait. But suddenly, I had time. I had necessity. I had nothing left to give—except to myself. And honestly, she was long overdue for some attention.

And for the first time in my life, I did.

That first round of chemo broke my body—but it opened my mind. And through that opening, light started pouring in.

Chapter 13: The Gift of Friendship

"A friend is someone who knows the song in your heart and can sing it back to you when you have forgotten the words." — Unknown

I have extraordinary friends. The kind you don't realize are quietly laying the groundwork for something beautiful until it unfolds in front of you like a lifeline.

Unbeknownst to me, my childhood best friend—the same miracle worker who connected me with the breast surgeon—had quietly mobilized an army of support. This behind-the-scenes operation would make a military logistics officer weep with joy. She pulled together a contact list from my bachelorette party, baby shower, and probably a few group texts I'd long forgotten about, assembling a team of friends from every chapter of my life: childhood, undergrad, grad school, various jobs, adulting. Most of them didn't know each other, but that didn't matter. She simply asked, "Would you like to help support Amanda over the next several months?"

Nearly everyone said yes. And just like that, she built a system—a chemotherapy cycle-specific support squad. Each group was "on deck" for a specific treatment round, like a coordinated relay team of angels with snacks and goodies.

Before every infusion, she would text me and gently ask what I needed, what foods sounded good, or what small comforts I was craving. Then, she'd pass the wish list along to that round's support crew. It was a stroke of logistical genius and deep emotional generosity.

And like clockwork, the day after chemo, care packages would arrive— full of thoughtful, tailored items. There were Spoonful of Comfort boxes when my mouth was full of sores, and soup was the only thing I could tolerate. Unscented lotions for my newly sandpaper skin. Cozy socks. Cute hats to cover my newly aerodynamic head, and electrolyte mixers for when even water tasted like it had a personal grudge against me. Loungewear so soft I wondered if it was woven by monks. These boxes didn't just hold items—they held intention.

What they gave me was so much more than what was in the box. They provided me with proof that I wasn't forgotten.

When you go through something traumatic, especially something prolonged like cancer treatment, the outpouring of love tends to come in waves. There's an initial swell of support after the diagnosis… and then, slowly, life returns to normal for everyone else. But your life doesn't.

Every three weeks, as my body was hit again with chemotherapy, their love arrived at my door. Their consistency reminded me that I wasn't alone. It's impossible to describe how deeply that kind of sustained support carries someone.

What made it even more special was the way my friend structured it. She gave people direction. She gave them a way to help that didn't feel overwhelming or uncertain. Many people want to do something, but they don't know what to do or say, especially in situations that are heartbreaking or uncomfortable.

She eliminated that barrier for them. Grouping people meant no one had to shoulder the effort alone. And for those with limited time or resources, it provided an opportunity to contribute meaningfully without feeling overwhelmed.

Some friends went above and beyond. Some checked in with texts or sent their own surprise packages. When I casually mentioned that comfort was my new full-time job, three friends independently mailed me the coziest outfits imaginable. That's how I met the Vuori Performance Joggers, which I proceeded to wear approximately 400 out of the next 365 days. (No regrets.)

Another friend mailed me a cozy stocking cap from the golf course where I first learned how to golf—plus a Grubhub gift card. Pro tip: If you don't live in the same town, send food delivery. Nothing feels more powerful during chemo than telling your parents, "Don't worry, dinner's on me," and then watching takeout magically arrive 45 minutes later like you're some kind of DoorDash fairy godmother.

My Sigma Gamma Rho sisters from undergrad sent the sweetest box of sorority-branded goodies, which transported me straight back to my 20s. And yes, let's address the obvious: this (pre-chemo) blonde-haired, blue-eyed Montanan pledged a historically Black sorority in college. Those bonds run deep—the kind where she'll pick you up at the airport at 3 a.m. with snacks and zero complaints.

Through all of this, I learned something crucial about how we show up for people in crisis:

Never say, "Let me know if you need anything."

It's well-intentioned, but let's be honest—no one in crisis is going to respond with, "Actually, yes—could you swing by with a lasagna, help me fold laundry, and give me a foot massage?" Not because the person is actually fine, but because receiving—*really receiving*—requires vulnerability, and asking for help feels awkward at best, impossible at worst.

Instead, ask, "What do you need right now?"

Even better? Offer something specific. "What day can I send you dinner this week?" or "Would cozy socks or a sleep mask be helpful right now?" Give specifics. Give options. Give permission to say yes.

Having one trusted friend coordinate it all was also a gift I didn't know I needed. It spared me the exhaustion of repeating myself or coordinating logistics. Toward the end of treatment, when my body was weakening and my energy was depleted, just managing one point of contact was all I could manage.

Now, let's talk about flowers.

I never thought flowers could be… triggering. Even though I appreciated the gesture and knew it came from a loving place, I struggled to watch them wilt and die. In that fragile emotional state, they felt like a metaphor for what was happening to me. My sweet mom caught on quickly. Every time they started to turn, she'd quietly make them disappear. One less visual reminder of decay. One more way I was lovingly protected.

This season showed me that support doesn't have to be grand. Sometimes it's a snack you didn't know you needed. A soft blanket that helps you sleep. A text that arrives at just the right time.

But most of all, it's showing up. Again and again and again.

And that's precisely what Amanda's Army did.

Chapter 14: The Silent Strength of Caregivers

"Too often we underestimate the power of a touch, a smile, a kind word… all of which have the potential to turn a life around." — Leo Buscaglia

When cancer enters your life, it doesn't just happen to *you*. It happens to everyone who loves you.

So often, the focus—understandably—is on the patient. The one receiving the diagnosis. The one undergoing the treatment. But one of the most forgotten groups in times like this is the caregivers—the partners, parents, siblings, and friends who rearrange their lives overnight to hold up the world around you while yours feels like it's collapsing.

Yes, many cancer centers offer support groups for caregivers, and thank goodness they do. But emotional and social support from family, friends, and the community? That often gets overlooked.

Overnight, our family did a complete 180.

My parents had built a well-earned retirement life full of friends, dinners out, golf games, and sunset happy hours. But suddenly, all of that came to a screeching halt. With my immune system compromised, our household had to operate under strict precautions. No more visitors, no more nights out, no more community gatherings. Staying healthy—for me—became priority number one.

But that safety came at a cost.

It was isolating.

And not just for me, but for my parents too. They didn't complain— not once—but I saw it. They were shouldering an incredible weight, quietly and without question. And it didn't help that so much of the outside world, even well-meaning friends, didn't quite realize the emotional and physical toll caregiving can take.

That's why something as simple as a neighbor's call turned into a lifeline.

One of the women in my parents' community called and said, "Can I set up a meal train for you? I like doing it and I'm really good at it."

She had no idea how perfectly worded that offer was. It hadn't even dawned on my mom to ask for help. Like me, she would've likely said, "Oh, we're fine." But this woman didn't make it feel like a burden. She made it feel like it was a favor to *her* to get to help us. And that changed everything.

We needed it more than we knew.

Caring for an 18-month-old is exhausting under the best of circumstances—let alone when you're also caring for your adult daughter undergoing chemotherapy. Twice a week, home-cooked meals would appear at our door, filled with love, nourishment, and relief. They didn't just feed us—they sustained us.

Meanwhile, my husband was juggling an impossible schedule. Since we were living in Southern California, far from his usual work territory, he had to split his time—working in Colorado or Arizona during the week and then either flying or driving to be with us on the weekends. When he arrived, he would take over parenting duties so my parents could get a much-needed break.

And then on Monday, he'd do it all again.

He never complained. But it was hard—especially for someone who's naturally social, whose friendships and energy come from being around others. So, when golf became the one COVID-safe outlet he could keep, it was more than just a sport—it was therapy. And the friends and coworkers who checked in on him, invited him out, or gave him space to just be "normal" for a little while? They were doing far more than they realized.

And then there was my brother.

As a PICU doctor, he has one of the most demanding, emotionally intense jobs imaginable. And yet, he grouped his shifts and call days so that he could fly in and stay with us for days at a time—often four days or longer. He didn't just show up—he showed up *fully*.

He was the ultimate playmate for my daughter. Their bond, forged in that difficult season, is unshakable. To this day, they're "best buddies," a title she gave him herself. He brought lightness into our home, laughter into our routine, and joy into our daughter's world.

But he, too, made sacrifices. He gave up his social life. Rearranged his work. Showed up for us when we needed him most. And his friends and colleagues who took on extra shifts or checked in on him? Their quiet support made it all possible.

It takes a village.

In our case, it took an army.

And yet, several nights I would cry myself to sleep—not just because of what *I* was going through—but because I couldn't stop thinking about the people who face this kind of battle alone. The single parents. The elderly with no family nearby. The caregivers who collapse from exhaustion, with no one checking on *them*. The people who lose homes because they can no longer afford a mortgage due to medical bills.

These are the quiet casualties of illness—the ones whose names aren't in the patient charts, but who suffer deeply just the same.

That's why nonprofits that serve these forgotten groups are true heroes. They step in where family, finances, or faith communities fall short. Their work matters more than most of us will ever know.

In all the darkness, that was the light: watching people step up for *my* caregivers. Knowing that love wasn't just coming to me—but flowing through me, wrapping around those who held me up when I couldn't stand on my own.

Cancer doesn't just test your body. It tests the people around you.

And our team? Our team passed the test with flying colors, demonstrating love, grit, and grace.

Chapter 15: Going Bald (On Purpose)

"What you lose can be replaced by what you find within." — Anonymous

Losing your hair is a strange kind of grief. It's not painful. It's not even necessarily surprising. But it's visible, like a blinking neon sign that says, *Hi, I'm in cancer treatment!* It's an undeniable marker that you're now living a different life—a patient life. A cancer life.

Early on, I learned about a method called *cold-capping*. The idea is to wear a freezing cold cap—literally, a helmet packed with ice or cooled with a machine—on your head during each chemo session. Think brain freeze meets medieval torture device. The extreme cold constricts the blood vessels in your scalp, reducing the amount of chemo that reaches the hair follicles. In theory, it helps prevent your hair from falling out. In practice? It's a long, expensive, uncomfortable gamble.

I did my research. I talked to the companies, read the testimonials, and looked into rental costs. It wasn't cheap, and insurance didn't cover a dime of it. The process also added hours to already long chemotherapy days, with staff needing to change the caps every 20–30 minutes for maximum effect. And it wasn't guaranteed to work—especially not with the particular chemo agents I was on.

Honestly, it sounded like torture. Ice cream headaches on steroids. For the chance of *maybe* keeping some hair that I wasn't all that attached to in the first place?

I passed—hard pass.

Besides, I've never been particularly in love with my hair. It was fine—shoulder-length, naturally blonde, a little curly—but never something I saw as "my best feature." When I was younger, straight hair was the trend, and flatirons weren't really a thing yet. So, my curls got wrangled into a bun. For over a decade, that bun lived on top of my head like a helmet of its own. Being bald couldn't be that much worse… right?

I knew the shedding would start around the two- to three-week mark after my first chemo. So, in true planner fashion, I decided to get ahead of it. About two weeks in, I went to the salon and had my hair cut to just above my shoulders—closer to my chin, really. It was adorable. I loved it. Truly, I looked like the kind of woman who says things like, "Let's circle back on that" and means it. I remember staring at myself in the mirror, thinking: *Why didn't I do this years ago?* The answer, of course, was that I never had the guts. Funny what cancer can push you to do.

That cut was the beginning of my shift in mindset. I made a quiet vow to myself to honor every stage of this process. I wouldn't mourn what I lost—I'd celebrate what was new. I'd welcome growth when it came, and in the meantime, I'd find beauty in every transition. And if things got weird? Well, at least I'd have good stories.

A week later, the real shedding began.

I was determined not to have *that* moment—you know the one. The scene in every cancer movie where the protagonist looks down in the shower and sees a clump of hair, then slowly pulls more out in disbelief and horror. I didn't need the drama. I needed a clean slate.

So, I made the decision: time to shave it off.

Who better to do the honors than my bald, bearded husband? Who better to shave my head than someone already thriving in the bald community?

Romantic? Maybe.
Symbolic? Definitely.
A good idea? Debatable.

Turns out he missed his calling as a barber. Or rather—thankfully—he *never* considered it as a calling. What he gave me could only be described as a "half bowl cut meets accidental crop circle." There were lines. Angles. Random patches. It was somewhere between "accidental buzz cut" and "kindergarten scissors project." And it was… hilarious.

We laughed—really laughed. That deep, can't-breathe kind of laughter that you need when your whole world feels inside out. Eventually, my mom stepped in to save the day. She's been cutting my dad's hair for years, and thank goodness for that. She smoothed it all out, and together we turned a potential meltdown into a moment—something funny, tender, and oddly empowering.

When it was done, I looked in the mirror and saw someone fierce staring back.

I didn't look like "sick me." I looked like a warrior. Someone brave. Someone who looked like she might ride a motorcycle and teach hot yoga on the side.

Honestly? I kind of loved her.

I took a picture and posted it. Not for sympathy, but as a signal: *I'm still here. I'm still fighting. I still have jokes—and maybe a future in edgy hair modeling.*

I was ready—for round two of chemo and for whatever came next.

Chapter 16: When Side Effects Met Soundtracks

"Where words fail, music speaks." — Hans Christian Andersen

After I shaved my head and declared war on despair, I thought I was emotionally prepared for anything. But with each round of chemo, the side effects didn't just return—they brought reinforcements. Like they had a group chat titled *"Let's Wreck Amanda,"* and every week, someone new chimed in.

But I wasn't going down easy. I came into every infusion like a mom at a parent-teacher conference: calm, respectful, but very ready to advocate. I asked about every sensation, every change, every detail of every drug. If a nurse ever dared to say, "That's just the way it is," I'd smile sweetly, tilt my head, and say, "That's adorable—but no."

One of the worst side effects for me was mouth sores. Tiny little demons- painful enough to make eating a struggle and drinking feel like punishment. And staying hydrated was non-negotiable when it came to flushing out the chemo. I'd read in one of my Facebook support groups that sucking on ice chips during chemo could help prevent mouth sores—essentially cold-capping for your mouth. The logic made sense: reduce blood flow to the area so less chemo reaches the cells in your mouth. It sounded weird, but also... genius?

Not so fast. The problem was, I'd been given Benadryl to manage potential allergic reactions, and it knocked me out like I'd been hit with a tranquilizer dart. If I were asleep, I couldn't suck ice. (That sentence will never sound normal.) I brought it up with the team and asked if there was a non-drowsy alternative. They hesitated. I persisted. They relented and tried a different drug. And it worked. I stayed awake, used the ice chips, and from that point on, the mouth sores were few and far between. That one win, small as it was, felt monumental. It reminded me that self-advocacy isn't just helpful—it's vital.

Speaking of ice— let's talk about the chemo "surprise guest star" known as numbness and tingling in your hands and feet. Mine showed up after round two, like an uninvited plus-one to the party. I'd read that cold therapy mittens and socks could help, so I gave them a shot. They were chilly (okay, *very* chilly), but not unbearable—and wow, they worked. My system: have the nurses toss them in the freezer when I arrived, then pull them out 15–30 minutes before the drip started. My genius upgrade? A heated blanket wrapped around the rest of me like a cozy burrito. The result? I looked ready for a *Sports Illustrated* spread… in the "Extreme Sitting" edition. All I was missing was a sponsorship deal from Yeti.

The Facebook groups I joined were also full of little hacks like that. People posted about everything from managing nausea to navigating insurance claims. But they came with a dark side, too. Many of the stories that were shared were heartbreaking—worst-case scenarios from people who were scared, isolated, or angry. And understandably so. But I realized quickly that scrolling aimlessly could take a toll on my psyche. So, I made a rule: I only went into the group with a purpose. I would search a specific topic, grab the info I needed, and then log off. No rabbit holes. No pity parties. Just the wisdom I needed to move forward, and if I had a helpful tip, I would leave that too.

As part of my emotional armor, I also made a strict decision to avoid negative media. That meant no news—none. It wasn't easy. I didn't want to bury my head in the sand, but I knew what I needed most was clarity, calm, and a mindset primed for healing. Constant headlines about violence, division, and chaos weren't going to help. So, I created a media bubble filled only with positivity, wisdom, and encouragement. And that's where audiobooks and music came in.

I couldn't look at screens without getting nauseous, and even printed pages made my eyes and head ache. But audiobooks? They became my refuge. Whether lying in bed, resting in the infusion chair, or driving back and forth to the hospital, I always had a story in my ears—and these stories mattered.

The Power of Vulnerability by **Brené Brown**

I'd actually read this years ago and was profoundly impacted—back then, it felt like she was handing me the blueprint to a more authentic life. But this time? It hit on a cellular level. Her voice, her humor, her fierce belief that vulnerability is the birthplace of courage—it all felt different when I was listening from a chemo chair, wrapped in blankets, stripped of my usual armor.

She talks about how real connection happens when we allow ourselves to be seen—messy, scared, and imperfect. That used to sound noble; now it felt like my reality. I didn't have the energy to "perform" strength anymore, and somewhere in the exhaustion, I realized I didn't need to. Letting people see me in the rawest moments didn't make me weak—it made my relationships richer, more honest, and far more meaningful.

This round with Brené didn't just inspire me; it gave me permission to live out what I'd only understood intellectually before: that vulnerability wasn't my downfall. It was my superpower.

Greenlights by Matthew McConaughey

McConaughey's memoir was a jolt of life. His stories were wild, unconventional, and sometimes laugh-out-loud funny, but what resonated most were his life philosophies. The idea of "greenlights"— moments of momentum, of permission, of divine timing—became a powerful metaphor for my own journey. He reminded me that even red lights eventually turn green, and setbacks are often setups for something better. His confidence, authenticity, and poetic soul brought me strength on hard days and lifted me when I felt like I was running on empty.

Think Like a Monk by Jay Shetty

Jay Shetty's teachings offered something more grounded—a practical guide to mastering the mind through the lens of ancient wisdom. The book taught me how to detach from toxic thoughts, create space for peace, and find purpose in suffering. His sections on fear and acceptance especially resonated. He framed adversity not as a curse, but as a teacher. And in doing so, he helped me cultivate gratitude and resilience—not just during treatment, but in life beyond it.

Becoming Supernatural by **Dr. Joe Dispenza**

This one became my nightly lullaby. I listened to it again and again—especially on nights when my body ached and my mind raced. Dr. Dispenza merges science and spirituality in a way that makes the mystical feel tangible. His focus on the mind-body connection, as well as energy and frequency, helped me deepen my meditation practice and truly believe in my ability to influence my own healing. When I meditated, I could feel my consciousness shift. For that hour or two, I felt no pain—just stillness, lightness. His voice became my anchor, and his teachings gave me a sense of power over what often felt uncontrollable.

Spare by **Prince Harry**

This book became a shared ritual between my mom and me. We listened to it together during the long drives to and from USC Keck. Harry's vulnerability, humor, and love for his family were endearing. Hearing about his loss, identity struggles, and search for meaning brought a deep emotional connection. We laughed, we sighed, we reflected. It made those otherwise dreaded drives into something we looked forward to. And on our final trip, we finished the book like clockwork. There was something poetic about that timing—one journey closing as another was just beginning.

Music wasn't just background noise. It was medicine in its own right.

And at the very top of that playlist? Florida Georgia Line.

Yes, really. FGL has been my favorite band since the moment I saw them live at Red Rocks. They weren't even the headliner—they were still the up-and-comers—but the second they stepped on stage, I was hooked. It was like musical sunshine. Their sound, their energy, their unapologetic joy—it lit me up. I've been to one of their shows every year since (well, pre-cancer)—dancing like a lunatic, singing every word, possibly overdoing it on the cocktails. Zero regrets.

Even during treatment, the FGL love didn't fade. When I was wheeled into an MRI machine and the tech asked what music I wanted in my headphones, I didn't even hesitate: "Florida Georgia Line," I said. "No music makes me happier." It wasn't a request—it was a prescription.

Even after the band split and Tyler Hubbard went solo (his own "Greenlight" moment, if you ask me), I stayed loyal. Because his songs? They hit deep. Uplifting, human, real. They gave me permission to feel hopeful—to believe that joy was still available, even from a chemo chair.

One song that especially stuck with me was "Undivided," his duet with Tim McGraw.

> "I think it's time to come together / You and I can make a change / Maybe we can make a difference / Make the world a better place…"

Those lyrics weren't just a catchy hook. They were medicine. A reminder that in a world that felt splintered—both globally and inside my own body—unity was still possible. Peace was still possible. Healing wasn't just a physical process; it was a spiritual one.

And weirdly, my connection to the Hubbard's didn't end there.

Back when my daughter was an infant, I stumbled across Hayley Hubbard's Instagram. She was posting honest, practical content about parenting—none of that perfectly filtered stuff, just real mom life. She looked adorable, even while sleep-deprived, and her calm confidence gave me hope. Then I saw she had created a baby feeding course.

I signed up for *Feeding Your Baby Solids* immediately—and I kid you not, it saved me. I was drowning in confusion about purées, feeding schedules, and what the heck a "baby-led bite" even was. Her calm, clear guidance tossed me a life raft.

We've never actually met, but I'm fairly certain that if we did, we'd be instant friends—the kind who finish each other's sentences and share snacks without even asking.

There were days when I could barely lift my head. I felt awful. Weak. Motionless. But I turned on that playlist, and slowly… I started to move. Just my hips at first. Barely perceptible micro-movements. But in my mind? I was front row at a concert—singing every word, dancing my heart out, living.

That imagined joy was real enough to get me through.

I'll never forget the night I actually had enough energy to give my daughter her bath. Most nights, I'd make it through dinner and then drag myself to bed like I was training for the Sleep Olympics. But this night? This was a gold-medal energy day. I wanted to keep the momentum going, so I decided to add music to the mix.

Growing up, my mom always had music playing in the house. It was the soundtrack to my childhood. Thanks to her, I can belt out most songs from the '80s and '90s—just don't ask me to tell you who sings them—my brain stores lyrics, not artist names.

When it came to picking something for my daughter, I decided to make it count. She was only a toddler, but it's never too early for some girl-power inspiration. And honestly, I don't think there's a better young female entertainer to look up to than Taylor Swift. She's talented, smart, a brilliant storyteller, fiercely independent, and somehow manages to balance glitter, grit, and grace all at once. She stands up for herself, supports other women, and writes songs that make you feel seen—whether you're sixteen, thirty-six, or in chemo.

Plus, her music? It's impossible to stay still. Even on my most exhausted days, a Taylor beat could make my toes wiggle in the bathwater. So, it became our ritual: on the rare nights I had the strength for bathtime, we rocked out to Taylor. My daughter splashed and giggled, and I sang into the loofah as if it were a sold-out stadium. For those few minutes, the bathroom was our little concert arena.

Amanda Gunville

In the end, those audiobooks and the music weren't just entertainment—they were lifelines. Each one offered a different kind of medicine: courage, clarity, joy, or connection. And together, they helped build a mindset that wasn't just about surviving cancer—but about growing through it. Because healing isn't just physical, it's mental, emotional, and spiritual too.

Chemo may have stripped me of a lot—hair, energy, taste buds—but it also gave me something too: a reason to curate what filled my head and heart. Music and stories became medicine. Not the kind you swallow, but the kind you feel. Not in your veins—but in your soul.

Because healing isn't just about killing cancer cells, it's about keeping your *joy* cells alive.

Sometimes that means ice chips.

Sometimes it means replaying *Greenlights* just to hear McConaughey whisper "alright, alright, alright" like a spiritual mantra or hearing Prince Harry's British accent.

Sometimes it means Brené Brown telling you that vulnerability is your superpower.

And sometimes it means dancing in your mind to a country anthem—even when your body's still wrapped in a heated blanket, surrounded by saltines and Gatorade—because you can still have a Taylor-worthy moment, even if your only audience is a toddler and a rubber duck.

Chapter 17: The Leave I Didn't Ask For

"Sometimes when things are falling apart, they may actually be falling into place."
— Unknown

It was halfway through my six relentless chemo treatments when the call came. My business partner—technically, my boss—reached out and said she wanted to talk. Her tone was gentle but direct. She thought it was time we discussed my taking a medical leave.

I shouldn't have been, but I was stunned. Numb. A wave of emotions hit me all at once—shock, anger, sadness, and resentment. Yes, I was sick. Really sick. But I was still working. I attended every video meeting I could, even when I could barely sit upright. I'd turned my bedroom into a makeshift office, complete with a pop-up green screen to hide the reality of my situation—my unmade bed, the medical supplies, the nightstand crowded with medications. I wore wigs or scarves to look "presentable." I pushed through the nausea, the exhaustion, the brain fog. I missed meetings sometimes, especially around infusion days, but I kept showing up—because working made me feel normal. It gave me purpose. And I didn't want cancer to take that, too.

So, when she suggested a leave of absence, unpaid, my gut reaction wasn't relief. It was devastation. I felt like the ground had shifted beneath me—again.

For three years, I had poured everything into this company. Not just time and energy, but real skin in the game: I had personally invested in every round of funding, as had members of my family. I helped scale the business into triple-digit growth year after year. We were becoming the official wine sponsor of the Genesis Invitational on the PGA Tour—a full-circle moment that united my two passions: wine and golf. I had championed the decision to build our own bottling line, a massive leap forward for the brand. The company was thriving—and I knew my contributions were a meaningful part of that success.

I had helped build something remarkable. And now, in the middle of the most vulnerable chapter of my life, I *felt* like I was being politely escorted out of the party I helped throw.

The decision was ultimately mine, she said. My job would be waiting when I was healthy again. The message was clear: step back, recharge. And as much as I hated to admit it, she wasn't wrong—I was basically running on 3% battery with no charger in sight.

I needed space to process. I talked with my family. I cried. I vented to my business coach. Slowly, clarity began to rise from the noise. This wasn't a defeat—it was a pivot. A reframe. Maybe this wasn't me being pushed out. Maybe it was the universe handing me a hall pass that said: "Sit down. Catch your breath. The game will still be here when you're ready."

So, I said yes. I accepted the leave. But on my terms.

There were two major events I had poured my heart into—one at the Genesis Invitational and another surrounding the BNP Paribas Open tennis tournament in Indian Wells. I wasn't going to vanish before they happened. I attended meetings, tied up loose ends, and ensured they went off without a hitch. At the Genesis, I made it through every single day—despite the fatigue, the constant bathroom breaks in the nearest outhouse, and the ever-lingering nausea. At the tennis event, I arrived in a wheelchair and a brand-new wig, determined not to let my circumstances define me. I wasn't ready to sit on the sidelines. I wanted to finish what I started.

This was my "Obstacle is the Way" moment—again. And like every obstacle before it, something beautiful was waiting on the other side.

Chapter 18: A New Door Opens

"When one door of happiness closes, another opens." — Helen Keller

Apparently, when one door closes... another one swings wide open, holding a perfectly poured glass of bold, velvety Cabernet and a vision board.

One of the silver linings came from a familiar and trusted place: a consulting client who had become a cherished friend. The founder of the real estate development company I'd been advising had become one of my greatest champions throughout my diagnosis. Her heart is as expansive as they come—empathetic, generous, and deeply rooted in compassion. The kind of person you want in your corner... and at your dinner table, because she pairs encouragement with the ease of a perfectly aged Cabernet—full-bodied, complex, and exactly what you need after a long day.

When she heard I was going on leave, she didn't see it as a setback. She saw it as an opening.

"If you have the bandwidth—and only if you *want* to use your brain this way—I'm here for it," she told me. "Let's dream bigger."

Before this, our work together had primarily focused on funding strategies and financial modeling. But now, freed from the urgent demands of my day-to-day role, we began exploring something deeper. We asked: *What kind of company do we want to build?* Not just financially sustainable, but culturally extraordinary. What would it look like to create a team where humanity came first, where wellness and impact weren't buzzwords but foundational principles?

We started sketching the framework for an ecosystem that honored people, purpose, and innovation in equal measure. It was some of the most inspired work I've ever done —part brainstorm, part therapy session, part "Shark Tank" without the sharks. Our conversations were rooted in abundance—not scarcity. Possibility, not pressure. Hope, not hustle.

In a season that had taken so much from me, this creative burst reminded me what I still had to give.

This leave wasn't just about stepping back from my old role. It was about stepping into a new kind of leadership —one that didn't require me to prove my strength by muscling through 14-hour days, but instead asked me to build from a place of truth. One where success didn't mean hiding the hard parts, but honoring them—and using them to build something better.

Cancer tried to take a lot from me. But it gave me something, too: the clarity (and, let's be real, the forced downtime) to reimagine the next chapter.

Chapter 19: Angels Among Us

"Coincidence is God's way of remaining anonymous." — Albert Einstein

There are angels that live among us—unseen forces of grace, compassion, and guidance who show up exactly when we need them. I met one in an elevator in Los Angeles, on the eve of one of my first chemotherapy treatments.

My mom and I had just checked into our hotel. I was dressed in the usual uniform of comfort—soft clothes, makeup applied carefully, and either a pretty scarf or one of my wigs. I didn't look particularly sick, not that day. It was early in the journey, and I was doing everything I could to maintain some semblance of normalcy. We wheeled our suitcases into the elevator, which already had a few people inside. Usually, I avoided crowded spaces—I couldn't risk unnecessary exposure with my immune system already under siege. But for whatever reason, we rode up with them.

One stop passed, and a couple of people exited, leaving just one woman with us.

She looked at me, then gently asked, "Are you spiritual?"

I was caught off guard. "Well… yes," I said, unsure where this was going.

"Do you mind if I pray for you?" she asked, her tone calm and certain.

I fumbled for words but managed, "Sure, that would be great."

Just then, the elevator dinged—it was our floor. The doors opened, and she stepped out with us. Then, without hesitation, she reached for both my hands and my mom's.

"Something deep inside told me I needed to pray for you," she said.

I swallowed hard. "Actually, I was just diagnosed with breast cancer. I have chemo tomorrow."

Without missing a beat, she closed her eyes and began to pray: "Heavenly Father, I pray that you heal Amanda from her head to her toes..." Her words flowed with clarity and purpose. My eyes filled with tears, then overflowed. It didn't matter who she was or what religion she practiced. Her words were a balm—warm, healing, divine. I felt an energy I can't explain pulsing through me. A total stranger had seen me. Really seen me. And wrapped me in the kind of love that goes beyond understanding.

That woman—whoever she was—was an angel. No wings, no halo. Just a kind soul moved by something bigger.

I've always said my mom is an angel walking this earth. She's the kindest, most giving person I know—her default setting is generosity. I often tease her that she needs to live to be 126 because I plan on making it to 100, and I can't imagine a single day without her by my side.

And then there was my massage therapist angel.

Massage has always been my favorite indulgence—but in my pre-cancer life, I treated it like a once-a-year guilty pleasure—somewhere between "only on vacation" and "maybe if I win the lottery." During chemo, though, I reframed it completely. It wasn't indulgence—it was treatment. My way of coaxing toxins out of my body, soothing muscles that felt like they'd been through a demolition derby, and giving myself something—anything—to look forward to the week after each infusion.

She was so sweet, with a calm presence and hands that could have made a brick wall relax. I could feel her pouring positive energy into me with every session, kneading hope right back into my body alongside the sore muscles. By the end, I'd leave her table feeling just a little more whole—like she had pressed the reset button on my nervous system. Honestly, I'm not sure if she knew she was part healer, part therapist, and part magician, but she was. And she never once made me feel like I was "just a client." I was a person she was helping restore.

Another angel in my life didn't appear out of nowhere. She'd been part of it for as long as I could remember.

She's an oncology nurse by profession, a lifelong family friend by bond. To my mom, she's like a second daughter. To me, she's like the sister I never had—fierce, loyal, and always willing to speak truth, whether I wanted to hear it or not.

Halfway through chemo—when things were getting darker by the minute—she sent me a video message. I was drained, physically and emotionally, barely functioning. She looked into the camera with her no-nonsense face and said, "Mand, here's what we're going to do…"

It was exactly what I needed—someone to take charge. Someone who knew what I was going through and wasn't afraid to lay out a plan.

One of the biggest lessons in chemo is *don't chase your symptoms.* The moment you feel nausea, fatigue, or pain—you treat it. Immediately. But I've never liked medication. I've always been the "tough it out" type. Other than birth control, which I only started after years of horrendous periods, I rarely took anything.

It actually took my brother to snap me into action on that front. During a visit, he noticed I was going to the bathroom every 20–30 minutes to change my tampon.

"Sister," he said, "I'm not a gynecologist, but this isn't normal. You're losing too much blood."

He was right. My OB had been telling me for years to start birth control to manage it, but I kept resisting—until that conversation finally pushed me over the edge.

So, it's no surprise I had been resisting some of the "optional" medications prescribed during chemo. I wasn't terrible—I took some of them—but not all. My nurse-angel friend changed that. She outlined a new protocol that emphasized sleep above all else.

"These meds aren't addictive," she told me. "They're not long-term. They're tools. You *need* sleep to get through this."

It made sense, especially because the steroids I had to take before and after infusions gave me a false sense of invincibility—and kept me wired, unable to sleep. But when the steroids wore off, the crash was brutal. No sleep made everything worse: the nausea, the pain, the emotional spirals.

So, I listened. I took the meds. I prioritized rest like it was my job. And the difference was night and day. At my next chemo session, I showed up rested and protected—a total shift. It didn't make the treatment easy, but it made it survivable. I was still in the fight, but now I had armor.

She knew exactly what I needed, and she didn't wait for me to ask for it.

That's what angels do.

Not all angels have wings. Some ride elevators. Some wear scrubs. Some work behind a massage table with magic hands. Some know you your whole life, and others you'll never see again.

But every one of them leaves a mark—one that reminds you that even in your darkest moments, you are not alone.

And sometimes, that reminder is the most powerful medicine of all.

Chapter 20: Manifestation, Meditation, and Miracles

"Once you make a decision, the universe conspires to make it happen."
— Ralph Waldo Emerson

After a while, I started wondering if there was some secret group text for angels—like they were all coordinating behind the scenes.

"Okay team, Amanda's got chemo on Wednesday. Elevator Angel, you're up Tuesday night. Massage Angel, you take the week after to undo the damage. Financial Angel—you're on deck for morale and mortgage duty."

Because just when I thought I'd met all the angels, another one appeared—this time wearing a metaphorical lab coat stitched from generosity and pure heart. He wasn't a doctor; he was my husband's college friend. He reached out with warmth in his message and said, essentially, *We've got you.*

When I lost my paycheck, I could feel the anxiety begin to settle deep in my chest like an anchor. Though I was lucky to still have health insurance through my husband, it didn't come close to covering the mountain of expenses piling up. Deductibles. Out-of-pocket maximums. Travel back and forth to Los Angeles for treatment. Hotel stays. Gas. Meals. Parking. It added up fast. And on top of that, our mortgage still had to be paid. Just before my diagnosis, we had invested most of our liquid savings—our safety net was gone.

I was terrified.

Once again, I turned to meditation. I needed to believe that the universe, or God, or something greater than me, could still provide. I began meditating on abundance. I visualized a healthy bank account. I whispered affirmations that everything would be taken care of. I imagined a safety net beneath us, even if I couldn't see it yet.

Then one day, the net appeared.

I opened a Facebook message from one of my husband's closest college friends. His mother had passed away from breast cancer years ago, and in her honor, they had created a foundation. I hadn't reached out. I hadn't asked. But he messaged me out of the blue:

"It goes without saying, but we are here if you need anything financially. Airline tickets, lodging. Lots of costs insurance won't cover—and you don't need any financial stressors!"

I stared at the message and burst into tears. My heart cracked open.

Still, it was hard for me to accept help, let alone ask for it. I've always prided myself on being strong, independent, and resourceful. But I also knew that pride wasn't going to pay for a plane ticket or keep our house during treatment.

I took a deep breath and responded:

"I want to thank you for your kind offer to help us. It's super uncomfortable for me to ask for help and makes me feel really vulnerable, so bear with me. I just found out this week that my work will not be paying me for taking a leave. Our company does not provide disability insurance, nor do I qualify for state disability.

I'm not sure how your amazing organization works, but here are the costs we're looking at that aren't covered by insurance... Please know ANYTHING is beyond appreciated! We love you and your HUGE heart."

His response was instant:

"We got you. There is zero shame in asking for help, and I'm so thankful you did! Thank you for letting me help! I'll mail you a check today."

It was the exact sign I needed. I had checked with all the major cancer foundations, but because of my specific circumstances—income level, location, insurance status—we didn't qualify for any formal aid. This gift from someone who simply cared, who understood, lifted the weight that had been crushing me. Not just financially, but emotionally. It reminded me that we were not alone.

A Home Away from Home

After six rounds of chemo, the next mountain was the double mastectomy. The surgery would take place in Los Angeles, and I'd need to remain close to the hospital for recovery, anywhere from four to six weeks. Traveling back and forth wasn't an option, especially for follow-up appointments and in case of complications.

I began researching short-term rentals in the area, but the prices were beyond our budget. I reached out to friends in Southern California, hoping someone might have a connection, a lead, anything. Nothing came together.

Then—another moment of divine timing.

My parents had been invited to dinner by some friends. They hadn't gone out in ages, but I encouraged them to go. "It's outdoors," I said, "You need a break too. It'll be safe."

At dinner, they were introduced to a couple from our hometown in Montana. Strangely, they'd never met, even though they had dozens of mutual friends. As they chatted, the topic of me—and my cancer journey—came up. My mom, who normally holds things close to the chest, opened up and shared our current struggle: the surgery, the recovery time, the impossible cost of housing.

She didn't know this couple had a second home in Newport Beach. She wasn't asking for anything.

Without hesitation, the woman said, "Stay at our house. We won't be there, and it's big enough for your whole family."

My mom burst into tears at the table.

When she came home and told me what had happened, we both cried—hard. It felt like the universe had cracked open just enough to let a miracle through. Once again, the power of manifestation and prayer was undeniable.

I had meditated, visualized, asked silently for help—and it had arrived. Not always in the way I expected. Not on my timeline. But always right on time.

I learned that asking for help is not a weakness—it's an act of courage. Accepting help is not shameful—it's human. The universe, God, divine energy—whatever you want to call it—shows up in the form of people who care, friends who extend their hand, and strangers who offer their homes.

Meditation gave me the space to breathe, to quiet the panic, and to tune into a deeper knowing. Manifestation helped me align with what I needed—abundance, rest, relief—and to trust that it was possible, even when logic said otherwise.

There's no denying it now: thoughts are powerful. So is asking. So is receiving.

And so are the angels who answered the call.

Chapter 21: Glass Half Full – Chemo Edition

"A good laugh heals a lot of hurts." — Madeleine L'Engle

When most people picture chemo, they think of the "big three": nausea, fatigue, and hair loss. And, yes, those showed up to the party. But tucked in between the harder days were some delightful little plot twists—unexpected perks I never saw coming. Think of them as chemo's way of sliding you a few bonus points in the middle of a tough game.

1. No hair… anywhere.
Everyone talks about losing the hair on your head, but the real gift? No more shaving your legs or armpits for over a year. Smooth, silky limbs without the razor burn. And bikini waxes? Cancel that appointment— it's like your body accidentally signed up for the deluxe laser package.

2. The portion-control superpower.
Chemo gave everything a lovely metallic tang—like I was licking a penny dipped in seltzer. I love food, and normally when something tastes good, I don't just stop at "full." I stop at "regret." But when nothing tasted amazing, I learned to eat for actual hunger, not joy. Consider it an extreme (and very expensive) portion-control program.

3. Long, luxurious showers.
Before chemo, showers were like a NASCAR pit stop: wash hair, condition hair, shave legs, shave pits, rinse, get out. Once that list disappeared? All that was left to do was stand under the hot water and let it rain down like I was in a steamy spa commercial. Men, I finally get it—you've been onto something all along.

4. Flawless hair days—at will.
Scarves for home, wigs for the world. Pop one on, 20 seconds flat, and

boom—red carpet ready. No bad hair days. No humid frizz. No "I woke up like this" lies—because technically, I did.

5. Makeup made simple.
When you don't have eyelashes or eyebrows, makeup gets… streamlined. Sure, you can still pull off a smoky eye if you're committed, but I went the minimalist route. A little blush, a swipe of lipstick, maybe a quick brow pencil, and I was out the door. Under five minutes from start to finish.

6. VIP treatment.
Restaurants, hotels, airlines—when people find out you're in the cancer fight, kindness often flows freely. Free desserts, extra snacks, seat upgrades. You feel a little guilty… and then you remember, yeah, I've earned this tiramisu.

7. Front-row empathy.
I thought I understood compassion before cancer. Turns out, I was maybe a 5 out of 10. Now, I don't just hear someone's pain—I feel it in my bones. It can be heavy, sure, but it's also one of the most beautiful gifts this journey left me: a deeper, truer way to connect with people when they need it most.

8. Built-in nap license.
Chemo fatigue is the kind of exhaustion you can't fight, and nobody questions you when you say you need a nap. Mid-morning? Fine. Mid-meeting? Understandable. At a family BBQ? Hand me a throw pillow.

9. A free pass on the small stuff.
Someone cuts you off in traffic? Whatever. Kids spill juice on the couch? Eh. Chemo has a way of recalibrating your "Is this worth my energy?" meter. Spoiler: most things are not.

10. Instant perspective.
Once you've stared mortality in the face, a bad hair day, an overcooked steak, or a late Amazon delivery barely registers. Your gratitude muscle gets flexed.

11. The habit cure I never expected.

This one's personal. Ever since I was a toddler, whenever I was stressed, concentrating, or even just zoning out in front of the TV, I pulled out my hair. I'll never forget the day I looked in the mirror and realized I had basically given myself a reverse mohawk—a bald stripe running down the center of my head. Over the years, I tried everything to stop: hypnotherapy, shower caps, tying my hands together, and fidget gadgets. Nothing worked.

Until chemo.

When my previously long blonde hair grew back, it came in brown and curly—and for the first time in my life, I haven't once reached up to pull. The verdict is in: want to kick a lifelong habit? Forget self-help books. Apparently, the nuclear option is chemo.

For those wondering how my daughter fared while Mommy spent more time horizontal than vertical—let me assure you, she was living her absolute best life. People often ask me how hard it was to have such a young child during treatment. Honestly? I think I hit the jackpot with timing. She was done breastfeeding and past the fragile infant stage, but still young enough to have no clue what was really going on. (Although the first time she saw my bald head, she gave me a look like, *"Mom, did you lose a bet?"*)

Meanwhile, her days were packed with grandparent spoiling—especially from my dad, who turned into her personal chauffeur. They cruised the neighborhood on endless golf cart joyrides, fed ducks like it was a full-time job, and hit up every park within a ten-mile radius. And because we're a golf family, she also picked up "essential" life skills like raking sand traps and filling divots. Forget preschool—this kid was basically in caddie training camp. Her life during my chemo months? Wall-to-wall fun, laughter, and love.

Chapter 22: Crumbs and Clarity

"Hope is being able to see that there is light despite all of the darkness."
— Desmond Tutu

At the very start of treatment, my oncologist laid out two possible paths for what would come next. If my body had what's called a "complete response" to chemotherapy—meaning all detectable cancer cells were gone—I would continue with targeted therapies, Herceptin and Perjeta. These medications carried few side effects and would simply be part of my healing maintenance plan for a few months, and then we'd all high-five and move on.

But if there were even a single stubborn cancer cell lingering after chemo, the road would be longer—and rougher. I'd need to begin a year-long course of a drug called Kadcyla. Fourteen infusions. One every three weeks. In my breast cancer support group, Kadcyla reviews were basically the Yelp page for a questionable restaurant—some people swore it was "not bad at all," while others said, "Run for your life."

So, I made it my mission—mentally, emotionally, spiritually—to avoid it altogether.

Every day during meditation, I placed my hand gently over my left breast and envisioned it completely healed. I imagined the cells clean and clear, bathed in light. I repeated my affirmations: "My body knows how to heal. My cells are restoring. There is no cancer left." I wasn't just hoping—I was aligning everything in me with that reality. I believed. I had to.

As I approached the final stretch of chemotherapy—the sixth and last infusion—I underwent another round of imaging: an MRI and ultrasound to assess how well the treatment had worked. I had weathered each infusion with determination, but this test? It rattled me. I hadn't been that nervous since standing over a three-foot putt in the state tournament with everyone watching.

Two days later, I was back in my surgeon's office, bracing myself for the verdict.

She walked in with a bounce in her step and a grin that immediately had me thinking, either she has good news, or she just found out she's sitting front row at a Taylor Swift concert. "I have your results," she said, almost beaming. Then, "The second tumor—the one with a different pathology that we weren't sure would respond—completely disappeared. We can't detect it."

I stared at her, stunned. Tears welled up in my eyes before I could respond.

She went on: "The first mass, which started at 2.7 centimeters, has shrunk to 1.5—and it looks like cookie crumbles. It's dissolving. I'm hopeful that this final round of chemo will be like a dog coming to lick up the crumbs."

We both laughed, a rare moment of levity in a long stretch of seriousness. My mind immediately pictured Cookie Monster cleaning up my cancer like floor snacks. It was the happiest I'd been in a doctor's office in months.

Still, the definitive answer would come only after surgery. Once both breasts were removed and the tissue sent to pathology, we'd know for sure: complete response or not.

So, I waited.

Patience has never been my strong suit. I'm like someone refreshing the airline app every 30 seconds to see if the flight's still "on time." But for the first time in months, I was buoyed by real hope—scientific and spiritual. I kept meditating. I kept visualizing. I kept believing.

Because now, more than ever, it felt like the healing had already begun.

Chapter 23: Bye Bye Boobies

"Some changes look negative on the surface but you will soon realize that space is being created in your life for something new to emerge." — Eckhart Tolle

I dubbed my surgery Operation Bye Bye Boobies (BBB)—because in the long, often humorless slog of cancer treatment, sometimes you need to name things like they're a reality TV spinoff. Scheduled exactly four weeks after my final chemo, it was timed with the precision of a NASA launch. I coordinated with the surgical scheduler like she was mission control, and my plastic surgeon was set to be there to place expanders—temporary placeholders for the reconstruction months later.

By this point, I was starting to feel good again. Really good. The fog of chemotherapy had begun to lift, and I got a taste—just a taste—of what it might feel like when this was all over. I had almost forgotten what healthy felt like, what it meant to wake up and not feel like I was made of lead.

The day before surgery, my mom, my brother, and I drove to the West Coast. It turned into one of those perfect days you wish you could bottle. We walked the beach with sand between our toes, indulged in massages, demolished enough sushi to feed a mid-sized rowing team, and laughed like we'd just discovered the meaning of life. They let me choose everything, and I did so with the strategic focus of a coach calling the final play in overtime. I called it my "banner day"—one last celebration before stepping into the unknown.

Up until then, I thought I had made peace with losing my breasts. I really did. Ten years earlier, I'd found a lump (which turned out to be benign cystic tissue), and back *then* the thought of losing them had wrecked me. They were full, natural, and—let's be honest—one of my best features. They made me feel feminine, confident, and, later, nourished my daughter for six months. I was proud of what they had done for me.

But as the surgery date loomed, I convinced myself I was ready to let them go. They had served their purpose. They'd had a good run. I was ready to hang up the jersey.

Or so I thought.

The morning of surgery was *supposed* to run like clockwork—but my veins had other plans. After several failed attempts, a lot of apologetic smiles, and me starting to feel like a human pincushion at a dart-throwing contest, they finally got the IV in. Consent forms signed, I was then treated to a steady parade of surgeons and medical students filing in like they were speed dating my medical history. I smiled, nodded, and held it together.

But then, without warning, a wave of emotion overwhelmed me. I began to cry—uncontrollably. It hit like a tidal wave: the grief, the fear, the letting go. I didn't know where it was coming from, only that it was very real and very sudden.

I'll never forget one of the young medical students. She quickly grabbed a tissue, handed it to me, and gently placed her hand over mine. She didn't say a word. She didn't need to. Her quiet compassion grounded me. After so much structure, so many protocols, her warmth soothed me, and I was again settled.

I was ready.

Modern medical science is truly remarkable. About an hour before surgery, a radiologist injected a special dye into my breast tissue. This dye travels through the breast and collects in the sentinel lymph nodes— the first place cancer would likely spread if it had made a break for it. During surgery, the team would biopsy those nodes. If they were clear, they'd leave the rest alone. If they showed cancer, they'd remove the entire cluster. This moment would determine not just my treatment plan, but whether I remained at Stage 2 or progressed to Stage 4 —a rare occasion where I had absolutely no desire to overachieve.

The surgery lasted about six hours.

As they wheeled me into recovery, still groggy and fuzzy behind the oxygen mask, I pushed through the haze and whispered, "Lymph nodes?"

The nurse looked startled. "What?"

"Lymph nodes?" I repeated, a little louder, more clearly.

A smile spread across her face. "They were clear," she said gently.

I smiled and drifted back to sleep.

While I was still on the operating table, my surgeon had called my mom to provide an update. She and my brother were walking near the hospital, trying to breathe, trying not to let anxiety swallow them whole.

"The surgery is going very well," the surgeon reported. "We got clean margins. And all lymph nodes were clear."

My mom's knees gave out right there on the sidewalk. She and my brother clung to each other, crying tears they didn't realize they'd been holding back. Tears of relief. Of *joy*. Of the kind of disbelief that feels like grace.

I was cancer-free.

Chapter 24: Advocate Like You Mean It

"Raise your words, not your voice. It is rain that grows flowers, not thunder."
— Rumi

When I was finally released from post-op recovery, a nurse wheeled me down the long hallway to the hospital room where I'd be staying for the next couple of days. As we rolled through the doorway, I glanced around and immediately noticed something I hadn't anticipated: two beds.

Two beds meant one thing—this would be a shared room. I'd be recovering from a major surgery, stripped raw and exhausted, next to a stranger who was undoubtedly navigating their own post-op fog. No privacy. Unpredictable energy. Unknown noise. My stomach dropped.

Well, I thought, *can't hurt to ask.*

"Is there any chance I could get a private room?" I asked, my voice laced with hesitation. I didn't want to be *that* patient—the diva, the demanding one. But if cancer had taught me anything, it was this: no one was going to advocate for me better than I could for myself.

There was some humming and hawing, a "we'll see what we can do", and then—just like that—they obliged.

I got my very own room. My *penthouse suite,* I joked, even though it was just another sterile hospital space. But it was mine. That tiny win felt massive.

I was in pain and starving. I hadn't eaten in over 24 hours, and now the nausea had subsided enough that hunger was back with a vengeance. But this was a teaching hospital—staffed with residents, fellows, interns, and medical students, all of whom were stretched thin. So, I waited. And waited. And waited.

No food. No meds.

The nurse kept saying they hadn't received the orders yet, which meant her hands were tied. I was in increasing pain, with a rumbling stomach and no relief in sight. My mom, always the gentle nurturer, offered a suggestion.

"Do you want to do a meditation?" she asked sweetly, knowing how much they usually helped lift my mood.

"No!" I snapped, sharper than I meant to. "I want someone to advocate for me!"

I grabbed my phone. My surgeon—an angel, truly—had given me her personal cell and told me to reach out if I needed anything. I hesitated. I didn't want to tattle on her team. But I was nearing my breaking point and about ten minutes away from gnawing on my hospital gown.

I started drafting a text. My brother, sitting next to me, leaned over and gently took the phone from my hand. "Let me help," he said. His background working with families in hospital systems had made him an expert in assertive yet respectful communication. He read it over, softened the tone just enough, and hit send.

Ten minutes later, a nurse walked in with my pain medication and a warm meal.

Mission accomplished.

Later that evening, I thought about how different it felt to be in the patient bed this time. Years ago, when my college best friend had a double mastectomy, I had stayed overnight with her in the hospital. I remember watching the nurses come in and out through the night, checking her vitals and administering meds. She slept fairly well. I didn't sleep at all.

So this time, I made a different call. I sent my mom and brother to a hotel across the street. "You need a real night of sleep," I told them. "If I'm tired, I'll rest. But if we're all tired, that helps no one."

They hesitated—especially my mom—but ultimately agreed. And the next morning, they showed up bright-eyed and energized, ready to take care of me. That was the right choice.

Recovery was not without its challenges. One of the worst parts was the IV antibiotics. They burned like fire as they moved through my already fragile veins. Hours later, a phlebotomist returned to draw more blood. I winced as he prepped the needle.

My brother stepped in once more. This time with a calm, confident voice, he asked some pointed—but kind—questions. "Is this blood work medically necessary right now?" he asked. "Her veins are pretty shot, and the antibiotics were really painful for her. Can you double-check?"

The man paused, made a note in the chart, and left to "double check."

We never saw him again.

Another victory. Another lesson in advocacy. Sometimes it takes a text. Sometimes it takes a conversation. But always—it takes your voice.

And I was learning how to use mine. Loud and clear. And with just enough charm to still get dessert on the tray.

Even if it was just hospital Jell-O in my so-called penthouse suite.

Chapter 25: The Long Road Forward

"Fall seven times and stand up eight." — Japanese Proverb

Recovery was a rollercoaster—equal parts beauty, discomfort, and emotional whiplash.

The first week post-surgery, I was soaring. My mom, brother, and I arrived at our friend's home, the one they had generously offered for my recovery, and it was nothing short of a sanctuary. The house was wrapped in calming blues and whites, with a backyard that looked like it had been ripped from the pages of *Coastal Living*. If healing had a mailing address, this was it.

And I'll repeat it for the people in the back: I would do ten mastectomy surgeries before I'd do another round of chemo. Surgical recovery, while no walk in the park, was far more manageable. The worst part? The drains—four long, clear tubes stitched into my sides, slowly collecting fluid from the surgical sites.

I decided to name them—Henry, George, Clarence, and Leonard. It made me laugh to imagine them as a gang of old grandpas, stubbornly overstaying their welcome. Every day, I measured the output with a small sense of ceremony, willing the numbers to go down so they could finally be removed. It took three weeks, but eventually the levels dropped low enough. The day the drains came out, it felt like being released from a bizarre kind of house arrest. Sweet freedom.

I had prepared myself for what I'd see when I looked down at my chest—and, surprisingly, I wasn't traumatized. I had studied mastectomy scar photos online in the weeks before surgery, the same way other people study vacation rentals or restaurant menus. And somehow, it helped. My chest no longer felt like "private parts." It felt like a battlefield. And I was the survivor.

I even showed my brother. The incisions were massive, and I needed someone to make sure they looked okay. As strange as that sounds, it gave me comfort to hear him say, "They look good. Really." Somehow, that made me believe it.

From day two, I started walking—slow, careful laps, five minutes at a time, three times a day. Movement meant healing. And as much as I wanted to push myself, I stuck to the rules: no lifting, no pulling, no shortcuts. (I'd learned the hard way that shortcuts usually take twice as long.)

I must have been quite the sight—shuffling around the pool in my robe and slippers, bald head wrapped in a bright scarf, surgical drains clipped to my pockets like strange accessories. I looked less like a recovering patient and more like an eccentric retiree who'd wandered away from her cabana in search of a margarita.

Unlike during chemo—when I struggled to stay ahead of the pain—this time I had help. My brother, in full big brother-doctor mode, made me a medication schedule and taped it to the nightstand. It was surprisingly effective. You'd think remembering a few pill times wouldn't be hard, but when you're in pain and half-asleep, even simple things become a blur. That little schedule was gold. I took every dose on time, even in the middle of the night.

For a while, it felt like I was winning. My body was healing. My energy was creeping back. I even let myself imagine the finish line.

And then the call came.

It was the pathology report. The final word. The real verdict. And just like that—I was crushed. I did *not* have a complete response. There were still cancer cells in the breast tissue they had removed.

It meant one thing: more treatment. A whole year more. Fourteen cycles of a stronger, more targeted therapy. Kadcyla.

The emotional blow felt eerily similar to the day I first heard the words: *You have cancer.* I sobbed—deep, guttural, ugly sobs. There was no positive spin to be had in that moment. I didn't try. I let myself sink all the way into the grief of it—the loss of the clean break I thought I'd earned, the finish line I thought was right in front of me.

Because I had done *everything* right. I visualized healing. I meditated. I walked. I endured. And still, here we were.

But I've learned that honoring your emotions doesn't make you weak. In fact, it's quite the opposite. As someone who spent a lifetime keeping her feelings bottled up, I was finally learning that letting them out was powerful. Healthy, even.

Once I had cried all the tears and allowed myself to mourn what I thought would be the end, I did what I always do—I got back up. The battle wasn't over. This next chapter would be twice as long, yes, but I wasn't the same woman I had been when this started. I was wiser. Stronger. More resourced.

So, I picked up the sword again.

Armored. Ready.

And determined to finish the fight.

Chapter 26: Kadcyla - The Why Behind the "Extra Year"

"Faith is taking the first step even when you don't see the whole staircase."
— Martin Luther King Jr.

When I first heard the words *"you need another year of treatment,"* my brain immediately filed it under *Failure, with a capital F*. In my head, it wasn't the next step—it was a setback. I had pictured myself crossing the finish line, arms in the air, tape breaking across my chest... and instead, someone handed me another race bib and said, *"Congrats, now do the marathon again, but this time uphill in snow."*

I now see it was something else entirely: *insurance.*

Kadcyla (T-DM1) is a targeted antibody-drug conjugate that combines Herceptin (my old chemo companion) with a chemo agent. Think of it as a molecular Uber—Herceptin drives the chemo straight into the HER2-positive cancer cells and drops it off like, *"Here's your stop, now destroy yourself."* It's designed specifically for cases like mine, where there was still residual disease after neoadjuvant chemotherapy (aka, chemo before surgery). Miraculously, this drug was approved by the FDA only six years ago for my type of cancer.

The science is impressive: Kadcyla reduces the risk of recurrence by 50% in patients like me. Fifty percent. That's not just a small nudge in the right direction—that's life-changing odds. The Vegas sports book would be all over those numbers.

Still, I couldn't shake the feeling that I'd somehow flunked Cancer 101. I had meditated daily. I had visualized my cells glowing with health. I had imagined them regenerating like an HGTV kitchen remodel— clean, fresh, better than new. And yet, here we were. But maybe... just maybe... the meditation *had* worked. Maybe it gave me the clarity and calm to *receive* the next step in my healing. Maybe this "setback" wasn't a spiritual contradiction, but simply a scientific continuation.

I've learned that these two can coexist: faith and medicine, mindset and molecules, hope and Herceptin. And in that place of "both/and," I picked up my new race bib, rolled my shoulders back, and kept going.

Chapter 27: The Missing Piece No One Told Me

"When we know better, we do better." — Maya Angelou

A few weeks later, at a routine follow-up, one of the oncologists on my team casually dropped a sentence that stopped me mid–sip of water.

"In decades of practice, I've never seen an invasive, triple-positive patient have a complete response to neoadjuvant therapy."

I blinked. "Wait—*what?*"

Apparently, this was common knowledge in the oncology world—like knowing you never talk during someone's backswing in golf—but no one had bothered to mention it to me before surgery.

If I'd known that *most* triple-positive patients don't get a complete pathological response, I could have saved myself the emotional free-fall. I wouldn't have felt like I'd failed some sort of final exam. I would've walked into that post-surgery pathology meeting braced for Kadcyla instead of mentally booking my *end-of-treatment victory trip to Maui.*

Instead, I had spent days spiraling—wondering what I'd done wrong, whether my meditation had "stopped working," and if my cells were ignoring the very clear memo I'd been sending them: *You are healed. Please act accordingly.*

Here's the thing: this kind of information matters—a lot. When you're in the fight of your life, mindset isn't just a "nice to have" like extra legroom on a flight—it's survival gear. And knowing what's typical for your diagnosis can be the difference between feeling blindsided and feeling like you've got a playbook.

Kadcyla wasn't punishment. It wasn't proof that my body had failed me. It was protocol. Standard. Expected.

And knowing *that* was its own kind of medicine.

Chapter 28: Shifting Grounds, Steady Heart

"You can't stop the waves, but you can learn to surf." — Jon Kabat-Zinn

The rest of my surgical recovery unfolded about as smoothly as one could hope when you're stitched up, taped down, and draining like a makeshift science experiment. When my brother flew home to return to work, my aunt stepped in without missing a beat. She was yet another angel in my growing heavenly roster of support. Every time we were in a bind—especially when we needed an extra set of hands to care for my daughter—she was on the next flight out. Always with a radiant smile, an infectious laugh, and a love so steady and deep, I could exhale just knowing she was near.

With more treatment ahead, we made a big decision: follow my parents to their summer refuge—our hometown in Montana. Yes, this meant transferring hospitals (again), onboarding a brand-new medical team (again), and explaining my entire medical saga to people who were meeting me for the first time (again). But the tradeoff? Emotional safety. Familiar faces. Trees I'd known since I was five. It was worth every awkward new-patient intake form.

The first familiar face was my "little sister," the angel oncology nurse—though not by blood, she may as well have been. She was thrilled to have me under her care and took the reins with a fierce sense of responsibility. She was the kind of woman who doesn't walk into a room—she power-slides in with a clipboard and a mission. Appointments were booked, my new oncologist looped in, and my first infusion was scheduled before I had a moment to catch my breath. She was a force of nature—the kind that sweeps in like a storm, only to leave a rainbow behind.

One of the first things she changed was simple but genius: she scheduled me to return a few days after each infusion for an entire liter of IV fluids. It was just saline—but to me, it felt like liquid gold. After each treatment, I'd walk in feeling sluggish, foggy, drained—and leave renewed, like someone had jump-started my battery. Why hadn't I been doing this the whole time? Where had saline been all my life?

I leaned hard into exercise, walking even when it felt like I was moving through quicksand. The more exhausted I felt, the more I knew I needed to move. The paradox of chemo: stillness made everything worse, but motion—even the smallest kind—gave me back slices of myself.

Around that time, I also began Letrozole, a hormone blocker I'd take for the next five to ten years. At first, the side effects were tough. I felt off. I told my oncologist, and he explained that the alternatives weren't much better. He asked how I was sleeping— "Not great," I admitted. He gave me a few suggestions, simple things to improve my sleep hygiene. And, somehow, like magic, the side effects faded. Sleep, it turns out, really *is* medicine.

I started working with a physical therapist to regain strength and mobility in my shoulders and arms. My personal benchmark? I wanted to swing a golf club again. By the end of the summer, I was back to hitting short irons—nothing fancy, just controlled, steady swings. It wasn't exactly Augusta-worthy, but it felt like I had reclaimed a part of myself. One shoulder stretch at a time.

As fall crept in, another decision loomed: where would I go next? Should we follow my parents back to the desert? Return to Colorado? Stay in Montana? Kadcyla was far gentler than my initial chemo, but it still hit like a sneaky hangover—just enough to keep you from functioning at full capacity, especially with a toddler in tow. I couldn't manage caring for my daughter alone for more than an hour or so at a time. After much discussion and soul-searching, we made the call to head back to the desert.

It meant starting over yet again—with new doctors, new nurses, a new system of care. I didn't know then what that choice would lead to. I didn't yet realize that the desert held not just the next stage of treatment, but a powerful set of healing tools and therapies—ones that would help me find my way back. Not just to health.

But back to *me*.

Chapter 29: Let's Talk About Sex, Cancer, and the Pelvic Floor

"To love oneself is the beginning of a lifelong romance." — Oscar Wilde

By this point in my treatment, things had finally settled into a steady rhythm. I had my protocol, it was working, and the sheer logistical burden of trekking to Los Angeles for every single infusion wasn't something I wanted to repeat. So, I decided to look for a local option in the desert. As fate would have it, the nearby hospital had just hired a new oncologist who specialized in breast cancer. My Montana oncologist called her, and suddenly I had a new quarterback for Team Amanda.

She was warm, confident, and wicked smart—the kind of doctor who makes eye contact like she's tuning into your soul, not just checking a box on a chart. And just like that, I was connected to a new care team—including a physical therapist who would soon become one of the unsung heroes of my healing.

Now, the PT I'd seen back in Montana had been great. But this desert therapist? She was something else. Every session felt like magic. Every session felt like I'd upgraded my body's operating system. I'd shuffle in like Frankenstein's less-coordinated cousin and walk out like I'd just returned from a spa weekend with my joints properly aligned.

One day, she casually asked, "So, how's your pelvic floor doing?"

I blinked. *Wait, what?* Was she actually asking me about sex?

I had been in treatment for over a year and a half—dozens of medical appointments, endless scans, and more conversations about my body than I ever thought I'd have— and not *one* medical professional had mentioned the words "pelvic floor," "sexual recovery," or heaven forbid, "vaginal health." Not one. To be fair, my sex life at that point was… let's just say "dormant." I was terrified of getting pregnant and being forced to make an impossible decision. Thankfully, my husband was patient, kind, and completely understanding—unlike many heartbreaking stories I'd heard in support groups.

But let's be honest—I wasn't about to let him take a lifelong vow of celibacy in his 40s. We got creative—a little scheduling, some mood lighting, a lot of laughter. Foreplay took on a whole new meaning when you're trying to work around surgical scars, hormone-induced dryness, and whatever fresh nonsense menopause was throwing at me that week.

Speaking of dryness… oh, the joys of menopause in your early 40s. I awkwardly asked my previous (male) oncologist if there was *anything* I could do, and he swiftly handed me a prescription for vaginal estradiol. Effective? Maybe. But safe for hormone-positive breast cancer? The jury was still out. My other doctors were split on it—some saying it was fine in low doses, others looked like I'd asked if I could take up smoking. I stopped taking it after a few weeks — mostly out of caution, and partly out of sheer confusion.

But the work with my physical therapist? That was a game-changer. Yes, it was uncomfortable—sometimes downright painful—but I was determined. She reminded me of the pelvic floor therapist I'd seen after giving birth to my daughter. I approached it like training for a sport: not fun, but necessary. My goal was to get back to my "fighting weight"—both metaphorically and, let's be real, literally.

Fast-forward about a year, and I stumbled across a post in my online breast cancer support group. A woman shared that, for the first time since diagnosis, she had hope. Not just hope for survival, but for intimacy, for pleasure. For feeling like a whole woman again. She'd seen a specialist at MD Anderson in Arizona who had walked her through a step-by-step sexual recovery plan. The post exploded— everyone wanted to know what she was doing, how it worked, and where to sign up.

I took it a step further: I made an appointment, which required becoming a patient there first (because cancer bureaucracy is just *so* fun). I added yet another oncologist to my team—at this point, I was practically collecting them like friendship bracelets at a Taylor Swift concert—and then I went to see the sexual health specialist. She was every bit the magician I had hoped for.

She was the *first* person to ever explain what *actually* happens to the vagina during chemotherapy and hormone treatment. (Spoiler alert: it's not good.) She talked to me like an equal, like a woman who deserved pleasure, not just survival. Honestly, I wanted to cry with relief. *Why isn't this standard practice?*

Her plan was simple, but structured:

- Use a dilator once a week to gently stretch the vaginal walls.
- Massage internal scar tissue with a bizarre-looking snake tool that, frankly, should come with a user manual and a shot of tequila.
- Apply Revere, a hyaluronic acid suppository, every 2–3 days to restore hydration and elasticity.

I followed her instructions to the letter. I was the valedictorian of vaginal rehab—diligent, curious, and committed to homework. And slowly… I felt a change. Subtle at first. Then undeniable.

There was sensation again. Comfort. Even occasional pleasure —real, human, joyful pleasure.

There was *hope*.

And while I'm still on that journey—and maybe always will be— it feels profoundly empowering to take back this part of my life. Cancer takes so much. But this? This I could reclaim.

And let me tell you: that kind of healing? Game changer.

Chapter 30: Where East Meets West

"The part can never be well unless the whole is well." — Plato

When I told my new oncologist about the persistent body aches, deep fatigue, and general lack of energy I was experiencing, she didn't just nod sympathetically—she handed me a solution. "You should check out an acupuncturist in town," she said. "She's an M.D. *and* a Ph.D."

Say no more. That's exactly my kind of practitioner—someone who bridges the best of Western medicine with the wisdom of Eastern healing. A person who can quote both peer-reviewed studies and 2,000-year-old medical texts without flinching. A blend of data and intuition. Science and soul.

My first appointment was unlike anything I'd experienced in a traditional clinic. Before I even sat down, she asked to look at my tongue. I blinked in confusion—*my tongue?* Apparently, your tongue is like the fortune teller of internal health. It reveals everything from inflammation to circulation to whether your liver is throwing a tantrum. It was oddly intimate and weirdly accurate. Honestly, it felt like my body was finally being heard—but in a language I didn't even know I spoke.

Because I was still in active chemotherapy, my oncologist drew a hard line at herbal medicine (she didn't want anything messing with the cancer-killing cocktail), but she gave me the green light for acupuncture. I'd had success with it before—when I injured my back carrying my daughter around like a sack of potatoes, just one session had brought me back to life. But back pain and chemo fatigue felt like different animals entirely. I was cautiously hopeful but not overly confident.

And then… it started working.

After just a couple of sessions, my body pain—especially that deep, cellular ache that chemo leaves behind—began to ease. The soreness that used to slow me down in the morning was more manageable. My energy started to climb too—not enough to run a marathon, but enough to hike—real hikes, in nature, on trails, breathing fresh air. Not on chemo weeks (let's not get crazy), but in between cycles, I felt just enough like myself to lace up my shoes and move through the world again.

Here's what I learned: acupuncture helps by improving blood flow, balancing the nervous system, and calming inflammation—all things that chemo tends to disrupt. It also gently supports the body's own healing mechanisms. My digestion improved. My sleep got deeper. My nervous system felt less fried. That tiny army of needles was clearly doing more than just making me look like a porcupine.

When my chemo treatments ended, we re-evaluated. My acupuncturist suggested I try a short course of herbal medicine to help restore energy, rebalance hormones, and kick-start my internal systems. "Even a couple months can make a real difference," she said, in the same calm tone you might use to suggest trying almond milk instead of cream. She wasn't trying to sell me on a lifelong supplement plan—just a reset. A tune-up. Something to get my body's natural flow back on track.

It wasn't cheap, but after everything I'd been through, the cost of *not* investing in my healing felt much higher. So, I committed to a few months of herbs and regular acupuncture—part maintenance, part prevention. Because if this journey taught me anything, it's that you don't wait until your body is screaming to listen. And if a blend of needles, tea, and ancient wisdom could help me feel more like myself again—bring it on.

Chapter 31: Ringing the Bell

"Celebrate every victory, no matter how small." — Unknown

The week had finally arrived. My final chemo.

It would be my 21st infusion.

(And yes, if you're doing the math, that's more than the standard. They threw in a bonus HP infusion two weeks after my double mastectomy—because why not add one more to the party, right?)

And once again, divine timing showed up right on cue.

My "little sis" oncology nurse and her family were visiting us for spring break. We took our kids to Disneyland—because sometimes healing looks like churros, roller coasters, and belly laughs under a blue California sky. Their joy was contagious. Their smiles stretched ear to ear. And for the first time in a long time, I felt something so expansive in my chest I thought it might burst open: fullness. Hope. *Life.*

The next day, the anticipatory nausea was real. As in, I could practically smell the saline and feel the drip in my veins before I even walked into the infusion center. I'd become Pavlov's dog, but instead of drooling at a bell, my stomach did cartwheels like it was auditioning for Cirque du Soleil at the mere thought of an IV drip.

People kept asking, "Aren't you so excited?"

And I was. Sort of.

I was excited to not feel like I had the flu every night.
Excited to stop scheduling my life in three-week chemo cycles.
Excited to maybe have eyelashes again.
Excited to play with my daughter without needing a recovery nap afterward.

Excited to start getting pieces of my life back.
So yes, *I was excited.*

But also? It was complicated. Because when you're in the thick of treatment, chemo becomes this strange safety net. You hate it—but it's also the thing fighting for your life. It's like your phone's autocorrect—constantly messing things up, but somehow still useful. Letting go of it felt a little like walking without a net. Or ending a relationship that hurt you but also, in its own strange way, protected you.

Still, I showed up.

My infusion nurse smiled and said, "Ready to finish this?" I smiled back, settled into the chair, and watched the meds drip into my veins one final time.

At the end of the infusion, something beautiful happened.

The nursing staff gathered around me. They welcomed my family and friends into the treatment area, and one of them read a poem aloud:

"Your day has come to strike the bell,
your shining heart has much to tell,
find much to toll this proud new day—
your treatment is done, you're on your way."

I stood up, hand trembling, heart pounding. I reached for the bell and gave it a gentle tap. Soft. Polite. Canadian, almost. I didn't want to disturb the other patients. But then I thought:

This was my moment.
I've earned this.
We've all earned this.
Maybe it's even inspiring to those around me.

So, I rang it again. Louder. Stronger. I added a little dance for good measure. The room filled with applause, laughter, tears—*joy.* A kind of communal exhale none of us realized we'd been holding.

It didn't quite feel like a celebration yet—not fully—because I still had to get through the post-chemo crash, the bone pain, the exhaustion, the brain fog.

But none of that could touch this moment.
It was a marker.
A milestone.
A turning point.
A war cry.

The bell rang not just for me—but for every person still fighting, every hand that held mine, and every ounce of strength I didn't know I had.

I rang that bell for *her*—the woman I used to be.
And for *her*—the one I was becoming.
And for all of *us*—the survivors in motion.

Because survival isn't a finish line. It's a rhythm.
And that bell was my first note back to life.

Chapter 32: Bloodwork, Breakthroughs, and a Different Kind of Cure

"Peace is not the absence of conflict, but the presence of creative alternatives."
— Dorothy Thompson

It was time to get back to "real life," whatever that meant now.

My husband had spent the past year and a half commuting nearly every weekend—exhausting himself bouncing between Colorado, Arizona, and California like a human ping pong ball—all to be with us. It was time to reunite under one roof that didn't require a travel itinerary. So, we packed up and moved to Colorado.

And because the universe loves a good plot twist, a fascinating opportunity popped up almost immediately. I heard about a brand-new breast cancer vaccine entering clinical trials—with a participating site practically down the street. The early data was jaw-dropping: zero recurrences over five years in previous trial participants. Zero. As in… none.

I was intrigued. Deeply intrigued.

So, I did what any overachieving cancer nerd would do: I followed up. Repeatedly. Relentlessly. Eventually, I got a call back, and—surprise!— I added another doctor to my growing list of oncology specialists. Forget friendship bracelets—I was drafting MVPs like it was Fantasy Oncology League.

And wow, was she impressive. My new oncologist was brilliant—sharp as a tack, quoting studies off the top of her head to support every recommendation. But just as importantly, she had that grounding, warm bedside manner I had come to rely on. It was another divine pairing. I needed a local team anyway for my quarterly bloodwork, and it felt like the universe had delivered.

As part of the trial screening, I underwent a full workup. Thankfully, my trusty port was still in place, which made the mountain of blood draws far more manageable.

That's when my oncologist suggested something extra—a cutting-edge blood test from Natera, called the Signatera™ molecular residual disease (MRD) test.

This is how it works: Signatera is a personalized blood test designed to detect even the tiniest traces of circulating tumor DNA (ctDNA) in your bloodstream—well before a recurrence might show up on a scan or via symptoms. It uses your unique tumor's DNA like a fingerprint to detect even the tiniest leftover cancer cells in your bloodstream. Basically, it's the FBI of bloodwork—quietly combing through evidence, sniffing out any microscopic criminals still hiding out. Basically, it's the most advanced way to ask the question: *Is there still cancer hiding anywhere in your body?*

And I was ready for the truth.

But before those results arrived, I got another call—this one from the clinical trial coordinator.

I was standing on the sand in beautiful Newport Beach, celebrating my best friend's 40th birthday. The sun was shining, casting a golden shimmer across the waves, when my phone rang. The nurse's voice was kind but direct: *"I'm so sorry, but you didn't qualify for the trial."*

I paused. Took a deep breath. Let the wind fill my lungs.

"Okay," I said. Calm. Centered. Almost Zen.

She was surprised. "Wow… you took that way better than I expected."

To be honest, I surprised myself, too.

Here's the thing—I didn't feel disappointment. I felt *peace*. A quiet knowing inside told me I wasn't meant to be in that trial. Even with the impressive early results, something about it wasn't meant for me. I believe in following those quiet nudges—the ones that don't always make sense but always feel right.

The nurse went on to explain that my extra-sensitive estradiol bloodwork also showed that my estrogen levels were still creeping upward. This meant my ovaries were waking up, and with that came a higher risk of recurrence. We needed to act—fast.

There were two choices:

1. Monthly Lupron injections to shut down my ovaries chemically,
2. Or surgery to remove my ovaries and fallopian tubes entirely.

I tried Lupron first.

Within days, the emotional crash hit like a tidal wave. The only way I can describe it is *postpartum depression on steroids*. The darkness was thick. I didn't feel like myself—I felt like a shell of me. I was supposed to take this injection every month for the next 5 to 10 years. But I had just fought my way back to feeling human again. I tried it for two months. I couldn't do this. Not for a decade. Not even for one more month.

I had come *too far* to go back.

So, I called an audible: surgery it was.

That's when my personal oncologist dream team really proved its worth. There was debate—of course, there was—about whether to remove just the ovaries and fallopian tubes (an oophorectomy), or to include the uterus and have a full hysterectomy. The opinions were split, as they so often are in oncology. After reviewing all the evidence and trusting my gut, I chose the oophorectomy.

One week later, I was back in the OR.

Everyone told me it would be a breeze— "just a quick laparoscopic procedure, you'll be back on your feet in no time." Ha. Not quite. I ended up with not one, but *two* post-operative infections. My recovery was rougher than expected. The hardest blow? I had to cancel my long-awaited trip to a weeklong retreat with Dr. Joe Dispenza— something I had dreamed about for years. I was heartbroken. But I reminded myself: healing doesn't always happen on a beach or in a meditation hall. Sometimes it happens in a messy bed with ice packs and antibiotics.

And then, finally, *it* happened.

The Signatera results were in.

Negative.

Undetectable.

Not a single trace of circulating tumor DNA in my blood. No microscopic villains lurking in the shadows. This wasn't just a scan or a guess—this was data. This was *proof.*

I had technically been told I was cancer-free after my double mastectomy, but it never truly felt real. How could I believe I was healed when I was still hooked up to chemo bags, still dragging myself through infusions? But this… *this* felt different.

This was a new kind of freedom. A molecular-level victory.

That night, we dressed up and went out to dinner—fancy dresses, clinking glasses, laughter spilling like champagne. It wasn't just a celebration.

It was a homecoming.

To my body.
To my life.
To hope.
To joy.

To *me*.

Chapter 33: Rebuilding from the Inside Out

"Don't get back to normal. Get back to better." — Unknown

The journey after cancer doesn't end with the last chemo drip or surgical stitch. Recovery—true recovery—isn't just physical. It's emotional. It's spiritual. It's rebuilding not just a body, but a life. And I knew one thing for sure: I wasn't going back to who I was before. That woman was strong and driven, but her habits—overwork, under-sleeping, always pushing, giving too much—living at that pace practically rolled out the red carpet for disease. She meant well, but her lifestyle wasn't sustainable. I had worked too hard to heal—there was no way I was going to let old habits write the sequel.

I remembered the story of a prominent businesswoman—an icon to many—who had beaten cancer, only to fall back into the same high-pressure lifestyle that caused it in the first place. The cancer returned, and the second fight was far more brutal. She swore never to return to that version of herself again. Her story stuck with me. It served as a warning and a guidepost. I'd fought too hard to simply bounce back to burnout. I didn't want my life back. I wanted a better one.

Over the past two years, I'd grown used to biweekly bloodwork just to qualify for chemo. But those tests were limited. They told you enough to greenlight treatment—not how well your heart, liver, pancreas, or gut were functioning. I realized that I didn't want to just survive cancer—I wanted to optimize my body so it would never have to face another health battle of that magnitude again.

So, I enrolled in Dr. Mark Hyman's Functional Health Program. Functional medicine, unlike traditional care, takes a systems biology approach—it examines the entire body, not just individual symptoms. This program analyzed dozens of biomarkers to assess the health of every major organ system. I thought I was doing well—I was hiking, mostly eating clean, and just a few pounds heavier than my goal weight. But the data told a different story.

My A1c was elevated—I was pre-diabetic. My cholesterol was off, and my inflammatory markers were higher than I wanted. That was a hard pill to swallow. Hadn't I just walked through fire and emerged victorious? Apparently, my body had not gotten the memo. I was frustrated, honestly. But I've learned something important about fear: if you lean in instead of running from it, it becomes fuel.

So, I did what I always do when something scares me: I learned.

The first real step I took was reading *Outlive* by Dr. Peter Attia. Well—*listening* to it, actually, which turned out to be the better choice. His voice, calm and grounded, carried me through some of the most important health education I've ever received.

I also had a random personal connection to Peter. Years ago, I was in a relationship with someone who was close friends with Peter and his wife. We had a few dinners together—casual, relaxed evenings. His wife was warm and lovely, and I instantly liked her. I remember one dinner vividly. Peter had cooked, and when dessert came out—something decadent and creamy, full of fat—he made a bold proclamation:

"Fat isn't the enemy. Sugar is."

Back then, we were all drowning in low-fat propaganda. His words lodged in my brain like a seed, quietly waiting to sprout. And now? They made perfect sense. He was miles ahead of the curve, even then.

That dinner came back to me as I listened to *Outlive*. His work is nothing short of paradigm-shifting. In it, he challenges the entire modern medical model, particularly our obsession with lifespan over *healthspan*. He explains how most of us are living longer, but sicker—and that by the time diseases like cancer, Alzheimer's, or heart disease show up, it's often too late to course-correct. The real work is in prevention. In optimizing the systems of the body *before* they break down.

He introduced the concept of the Four Horsemen—heart disease, cancer, neurodegenerative disease, and metabolic dysfunction—and framed them not as inevitabilities, but as outcomes we can delay or even prevent with the right strategies. He talked about zone 2 cardio, VO2 max, strength training, and detailed insights into the metabolic processes most of us never think about but depend on every day.

But it wasn't just the science that moved me. It was knowing the integrity behind it. I had watched, years ago, as Peter quietly lived what he preached long before it was mainstream. That memory gave me even more confidence in his research. I trusted him.

So, I took notes. I bought the physical book so I could highlight, underline, and return to the sections that resonated the most. Yes, I was becoming a wellness nerd. It was the beginning of a new chapter—not just in learning, but in *unlearning* the habits and assumptions that no longer served me.

And somewhere in the back of my mind, I heard his voice from that dinner table again:
Fat isn't the enemy. Sugar is.

This time, I understood just how right he was.

Next, I read *Young Forever* by Dr. Mark Hyman, which perfectly complemented Dr. Attia's work. If Attia offered the "why," Hyman gave the "how." His message was deceptively radical: aging, at least the fast, painful decline we've been conditioned to accept, is not inevitable. Instead of resigning ourselves to arthritis, memory loss, and brittle bones, he argued we can influence the way we age at the cellular level—literally turning back some of the biological clocks we didn't even know were ticking.

Hyman broke it down into practical tools. He explained how our bodies have built-in detox pathways that work like housekeeping crews—if we nourish them properly. He dove deep into the microbiome, reminding me that gut health isn't just about digestion, it's about mood, immunity, and even long-term disease risk. He detailed how micronutrient imbalances silently chip away at our energy, and how chronic inflammation—this "silent fire"—isn't just uncomfortable, it's the root driver of nearly every disease of aging.

And unlike a lot of health books that feel like a lecture, *Young Forever* read like an owner's manual you actually want to open. Hyman painted a picture of aging not as decline, but as an opportunity to extend vitality, strength, and joy far beyond what most of us imagine possible. It wasn't about living forever, but about living *well* for as long as possible.

For me, his words were a relief. Attia had shown me the stakes; Hyman handed me the playbook. And for a recovering Type A like me, a roadmap of action steps—what to eat, how to move, when to rest—was pure catnip. It gave me the sense that I wasn't powerless against time or cancer. I had tools.

And so I turned my recovery into a self-experiment. I'd test an intervention for two months, then redo my labs.

Phase One: Sauna + Hiking.
It felt amazing. I sweat like a champ and had A+ mental clarity. But my numbers barely budged.

Phase Two: Supplements.
I tried them all—probiotics, heart health, anti-inflammatories, blood sugar stabilizers. But the nausea was real. I pared back to the essentials: vitamin K blend to prevent osteoporosis (common in women with breast cancer), a multivitamin with magnesium, vitamin D, omega-3s, and a mitochondrial support blend. A small uptick in improvement, but not transformative.

Phase Three: Strength + Cardio.
With a dedicated online program, I committed to a balanced regimen. My weight stayed the same, likely due to muscle gain, but my waistline refused to cooperate. Then, in a moment of hubris, I overdid it—and injured my back. Injury: one. Me: zero.

So, I pivoted.

Phase Four: Metabolic Reset with the Fast Metabolism Diet.
I'd used it in my 30s and it worked like a charm. Could it still help now, post-menopause, and with no HRT? I stuck to the plan precisely, eating the same meals I once had. Miraculously, it worked again. I shed the stubborn 10 pounds in 28 days with only walking and stretching. It was empowering.

Now I'm putting it all together: targeted exercise, foundational supplements, mindful eating. And the best part? My latest round of bloodwork finally showed a decrease in my A1C—a huge victory after all the effort I've put in. My lipids, on the other hand, are proving to be a little more stubborn. But that just means I need to stay consistent, diligent, and keep showing up. Progress is progress, and this win reminds me that change is happening—even if it comes one marker at a time.

But healing wasn't just about bloodwork and meal prep.

I dove deeper emotionally and spiritually. Meditation helped, but I needed more.

At MD Anderson, I worked with a clinical psychologist who specialized in post-cancer care. She helped me unpack grief and identity—especially around femininity. Cancer had stripped me of the physical symbols of womanhood: my hair, my lashes, my breasts, my reproductive organs.

"When was the last time you felt sexy?" she asked me once.

I laughed. "Definitely pre-cancer."

She wasn't amused.

"You need to reclaim that. Do your hair. Wear lipstick. Dress up even if you're going nowhere. Don't wait to feel better—dress like you already do."

So, I did. Slowly. At first, it felt silly. Then, it started to feel powerful. Dates with my husband. Solo moments with lipstick. Self-care became more than just bubble baths—it was a form of defiance. It said, "I'm still here. And I still sparkle."

Through a friend, I was also introduced to an energy worker who used hypnotherapy and guided meditation. Yes, it sounded woo-woo at first, but the effect was anything but. Her voice became my internal soundtrack. I listened daily. Her recordings didn't just soothe me—they *reprogrammed* me.

She taught me to visualize the future I wanted: vibrant, grounded, joyful. Not just free from illness—but full of life. I believed her. And eventually, I believed *me*.

After two straight years of treatments, surgeries, and more hospital gowns than actual outfits, my social life and travel calendar looked… well, let's just say even my passport had abandonment issues. My love language is Acts of Travel, and my cup wasn't just empty—it was clinking around with a sad little ice cube in the bottom. So, when January rolled around, I declared this *The Year of JSY*—Just Say Yes. Yes to travel. Yes to adventure. Yes to friend time. Yes to self-care. Yes to anything that didn't involve a waiting room, IV pole, or gown that tied in the back.

And let me tell you, JSY did not disappoint. Our family hopped a plane to Europe, and it was the first time I had been there since college graduation. I instantly wondered why I'd waited so long. I ate at restaurants so good I briefly considered changing careers to Michelin Star Judge—is that even a real job, or just my dream gig? I played golf (translation: took a nice walk, occasionally chased a small white ball, and decided not to care when the "walk" part was the highlight). I soaked up time with girlfriends, because nothing—and I mean *nothing*—recharges you like deep, soul-filling conversations with women who get you, preferably over wine and carbs. I saw my Notre Dame Fighting Irish play—yes, we lost, but no, I am *not* bad luck. And I laughed—a lot. The kind of deep, from-the-gut belly laughs that are almost as healing as any prescription.

Cancer didn't break me. It broke me *open*. What I've rebuilt since isn't just a body—it's a blueprint for a life I truly want to live.

This journey has reshaped every part of me—my body, my mind, and my spirit. Cancer tried to take everything, but in the end, it gave me something I never expected: a deeper understanding of myself and a profound respect for life. I now live with intention, curiosity, and fierce devotion to my well-being. I've learned to listen to my body like never before, to advocate for myself, to question everything, and to never mistake surviving for living. I am not the woman I was before cancer—I am stronger, softer, wiser, and more awake. And while I can't control what the future holds, I now walk into each day knowing I've done everything I can to live well, love fully, and leave nothing on the table. This is not the end of my story—it's the beginning of the one I was always meant to tell.

So, welcome. You are not alone. Make this the story you were always meant to tell...

Epilogue

"Get squished!" — Amanda Gunville

When I shared my diagnosis with the world, I closed with a simple PSA: *"Ladies my age—do not delay your mammogram."* Since then, I've basically turned into the self-appointed spokeswoman for boobies everywhere. I've told friends, family, and the occasional woman in the checkout line, *"Get them squished."* Subtle? No. Effective? Absolutely.

And here's why: I've already seen the impact. I've lost count of how many women have told me, *"I went because of you."* But my favorite story will always be my best friend's. After her mammogram, she was told, *"Just dense tissue, nothing to worry about."* But she pushed back: *"My best friend just went through breast cancer. I want to be sure."* Because she insisted, she got the MRI, the biopsy, and ultimately a lumpectomy. Since she caught it so early, her doctors determined she didn't need further treatment. That's not just a win, that's a confetti-cannon, champagne-toast, standing-ovation win.

I joke with her that I saved her life, but the truth is, she saved it herself by advocating for more answers. And that's the kind of ending I want for every woman. Not everyone can avoid cancer, but we *can* give ourselves the gift of early detection. And maybe, just maybe, that reminder you needed was tucked right here, in these pages.

So, here's your final nudge. Your gentle shove, wrapped in love and maybe a little sass: if you've been putting off your mammogram, go schedule it. Do it for yourself, for the people who love you, and for the chance to live long enough to find joy in every ridiculous, wonderful corner of life.

Because sometimes joy looks like laughter, or golf cart rides, or Taylor Swift dance parties in the bathtub. And sometimes joy looks like peace of mind—knowing you caught something early.

Either way, you deserve both.

Now go get squished… and then treat yourself to tacos, and maybe a margarita. Doctor's orders.

My Cancer Resource Playbook

After Diagnosis

1. **Get a second opinion.** If you feel even a flicker of doubt about your treatment plan, seek another opinion. Yes, it takes time and paperwork, but peace of mind is worth its weight in gold.
2. **Check out the books I mention in this memoir.** They may not change your life in the exact way they did mine, but I promise you'll pull at least one gem of wisdom from them.
3. **Schedule counseling.** For yourself, your relationship, your family—all of it. You are in a relationship with yourself, too, and that one needs support just as much as the others.
4. **Find a sexual health practitioner early.** I waited too long and wish I had started right away. Don't overlook this—it matters.
5. **Research cold capping.** I didn't do it, but many of my friends did and were glad they did. Look into it and decide what's right for you.
6. **Do a fun haircut.** If you're not cold-capping, think of this as your "audition" for every style you've ever wanted to try. Document it. Have fun with it.
7. **Buy a heated blanket.** Infusions are cold, and if you're also freezing your hands and feet with cold therapy, you'll want the cozy balance.
8. **Get cold therapy socks and mittens.** Not glamorous, but they can help minimize neuropathy. Pair them with that heated blanket—it's a vibe.
9. **Stock up on goodies.** Ginger chews, hydration mixes, protein bars, and whatever makes you smile. Little comforts matter.
10. **Buy cozy headscarves.** Wigs are wonderful, but scarves? Surprisingly stylish, lightweight, and comfy. I grew to love them.
11. **Download joy.** Your favorite playlists, audiobooks, or movies. Something that makes you laugh or relax. It passes the time and makes the IV beep feel like a finish line.

12. **Tell your people what you need.** They're not mind-readers. Be direct, and they'll be grateful for the guidance.
13. **Be vulnerable.** It's okay to not be okay. Honesty draws people closer—it's one of the unexpected gifts of this whole messy ride.

Day of Chemo

14. **Apply Lidocaine early.** At least 1–1.5 hours before your port is accessed. Plastic wrap on top, not gauze—trust me on this one.
15. **Move your body beforehand.** There's science behind it, but take it from me: I always felt better after exercising before chemo than when I didn't.
16. **Fuel up.** Even with nausea, try to give your body some fuel. Listen to what it needs.
17. **Chew ice chips.** Not glamorous, but a game-changer for preventing mouth sores.
18. **Bring a cooler for your cold booties and mittens.** Ask the nurses to pop them in the freezer when you arrive. You'll thank yourself.
19. **Advocate for yourself.** If something feels off, ask. You're not being "difficult"—you're being smart.

Recovery

20. **Be kind to yourself.** You've just been through a war. Take the nap. Wear the comfy clothes. Order the takeout.
21. **Prioritize sleep.** Rest, rest, and rest again. Ask for help from your medical team if sleep is hard to come by.
22. **Stay ahead of symptoms.** Don't wait for nausea, pain, or diarrhea to hit hard. Take your meds at the first sign. This is not the time to play hero.
23. **Hydrate like it's your job.** Water may taste awful—mine did—but keep experimenting until you find something that works.
24. **Get extra fluids.** A few days after infusion, go back in and ask for an extra liter of IV fluids. I resisted this for a long time because, honestly, who wants *another* appointment? But trust

me—total game changer. I'd walk in feeling sluggish and foggy, and walk out like someone had just jump-started my battery.

25. **Walk.** Even if it's just to the mailbox, it counts. And some days, it'll feel like crossing a marathon finish line. Celebrate it.
26. **Massage.** Once a luxury, now a recovery tool. It helps flush toxins and gives you something lovely to look forward to.
27. **Acupuncture.** I discovered it midway through and was amazed at the relief it brought. Worth exploring.

Surgery

28. **Write down a pain management schedule.** Post-surgery brain is foggy—trust the paper, not your memory.
29. **Find a physical therapist.** Especially one with post-mastectomy expertise. Commit to the program—you'll be glad you did.
30. **Move your body—gently, from day one.** Even if it's just standing up and shuffling a few steps, movement is part of healing right away. Start with tiny walks in your room or around your yard. Each day you'll go a little further, and those short strolls add up to real progress.
31. **Follow instructions.** This is not the time to be an overachiever. No lifting, no shortcuts. This is your chance to let others wait on you—say yes to it.

Final thought: Healing isn't linear, and it definitely doesn't come with a manual. These resources are simply the things that helped me most—little lifelines along the way. Take what fits, leave what doesn't, and know that you're not alone.

Visit hopeandjoy.net/resources for additional helpful tips and links to my favorite products.

Acknowledgments

To my husband, Jeff — thank you for walking this journey of life with me and for believing in me, even when it meant supporting my dream instead of me getting a "real" job. This book exists because you believed in us.

To my sweet baby, Jules — you are the light of our lives and our reason for being. You are my little miracle, and I can't wait to see the incredible impact you will make on this world. I love you to infinity and beyond.

To my parents, Fred and Laurie — my true heroes and unwavering support system. Without you, this road would have been far rougher, filled with giant potholes instead of just a few bumps. "Thank you" will never be enough.

To my big brother, Cam — thank you for being my lifelong protector and my greatest champion. Your love and energy for Jules is the greatest gift you could ever give me. I love you more than words could ever express.

To my Aunt Susan — thank you for saying "yes" every time we asked for your help. Your calm and joyful spirit was exactly what we needed. I cherish all of our heart-to-heart conversations, and I love you dearly.

To Kitty, my dearest friend — your steadfast support through every big moment in my life is nothing short of miraculous. Thank you for finding my life-saving surgeon and for organizing my army when I couldn't. I don't know what I did to deserve you, but I am endlessly grateful.

To Sung, my best friend — you've taught me more about life than I could ever count. Your loyalty is unmatched, and your friendship is a gift I'll treasure forever. You are my sister, and I love you deeply. Your dedication to helping guide and grow this mission ensures that the hope and joy born from my journey will reach far beyond me.

To my sweet Cass — your passion and knowledge made my journey so much lighter. The oncology world is lucky to have you, and I am lucky to have been loved by you — not just me, but my mom and my daughter, too.

To Eden, my devoted friend — thank you for years of friendship and for standing beside me as I carry this mission to spread hope and joy to the world.

To Jessa, my incredible visionary partner — thank you for showering me with love and endless positive affirmations. You keep my mind sharp and my heart full of abundance. You gave me purpose in a time when I could've felt forgotten.

To Amanda's Army — you will never fully understand the magnitude of the impact you had on my life. Through every high and low, you made me feel loved and never forgotten. I will forever hold you in my heart.

To Clint and Barb, our dear friends — your house was a gift from God and provided the healing sanctuary that I'll be endlessly grateful for.

To CA, our friend with a heart of gold — thank you for your generosity and for throwing us a lifeline when we needed it most.

To Cynthia and David — your care packages were next-level, from the custom hats to the bonsai tree. Every gesture made me feel loved. And allowing me to use your sound booth to record my audiobook — that generosity is beyond measure.

To Elise, our dear neighbor — you brought our community together with meals and love when we needed it most. Thank you for knowing exactly what to say and for making our lives a little easier during such a difficult time.

To Dr. Nelson, my breast surgeon — your positive energy and meticulous attention to detail are rare gifts to the world and to all of us warriors lucky enough to be in your care.

To my incredible team of oncologists, nurses, therapists, and counselors — your passion for what you do is inspiring. You are the unsung heroes in this world. I don't know how you do what you do, but I'm eternally grateful.

www.ingramcontent.com/pod-product-compliance
Lightning Source LLC
Chambersburg PA
CBHW031424120626
46545CB00006B/2270